T0107390

The I'M POSSIBLE Journey

Learning to Live with Sugar Addiction

Maureen Aliprandi

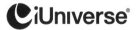

THE I'M POSSIBLE JOURNEY
LEARNING TO LIVE WITH SUGAR ADDICTION

Copyright © 2016 Maureen Aliprandi.

All rights reserved. No part of this book may be used or reproduced by any means, graphic, electronic, or mechanical, including photocopying, recording, taping or by any information storage retrieval system without the written permission of the author except in the case of brief quotations embodied in critical articles and reviews.

iUniverse books may be ordered through booksellers or by contacting:

iUniverse
1663 Liberty Drive
Bloomington, IN 47403
www.iuniverse.com
1-800-Authors (1-800-288-4677)

Because of the dynamic nature of the Internet, any web addresses or links contained in this book may have changed since publication and may no longer be valid. The views expressed in this work are solely those of the author and do not necessarily reflect the views of the publisher, and the publisher hereby disclaims any responsibility for them.

Any people depicted in stock imagery provided by Thinkstock are models, and such images are being used for illustrative purposes only.
Certain stock imagery © Thinkstock.

ISBN: 978-1-4917-8462-4 (sc)
ISBN: 978-1-4917-8461-7 (e)

Library of Congress Control Number: 2016900889

Print information available on the last page.

iUniverse rev. date: 03/01/2019

In memory of my dad.

John H. McCracken

An example and an encourager.

With grateful acknowledgment to family and friends who continue to encourage me with love, support, and feedback with no sugar added. And in appreciation for my readers. I wish you all the best.

CONTENTS

THIS IS NOT A DIET

It's a Do It

I've proven it oft: Diets really don't work.
I feel quite deprived and then go berserk!
I focus on numbers and not how I feel.
The scale starts to threaten and over I keel.
I throw up my hands with a "What is the use?
Why can't I get my clothes to feel loose?"

And then I just stopped. You could say on a dime,
But reality was a new paradigm!
The key to my health, and possible wealth:
Awareness of sugar and all of its stealth!

It's being aware of what to beware.
Having power. I'm able to care.
I write down my food, then pen my mood.
And follow the feeling with gratitude.

I remember hearing a dietician say to lose weight all one has to do is make
sure the calories in are fewer than the calories out. Easy as pie—or not.

I struggled with diets and weight gain and loss again and again for years
until I stopped trying to diet and instead began to focus my intentions
and energy on feeling better. The shift in my approach came after I
saw a book that suggested my mind and body troubles could be from
sensitivity to sugar.

"You're not lazy, self-indulgent, or undisciplined. Many people who
suffer from sugar sensitivity don't even know it—and they continue to
consume large quantities of sweets, breads, pasta, or alcohol. These
foods can trigger exhaustion or low self-esteem, yet their biochemical
impact makes those who are sugar sensitive crave them even more.
This vicious cycle can continue for years, leaving sufferers overweight,

fatigued, depressed, and sometimes alcoholic." (*Potatoes Not Prozac*, Kathleen DesMaisons, PhD)

I stumbled upon *Potatoes Not Prozac* completely by chance, but as soon as I began reading the cover, I suspected that this book had been written about me. The back of the book provided a spark of hope that was enough to ignite a quest to gain control of my physical and mental health. I wasn't an alcoholic, but I most certainly was a sugarholic. I had the other symptoms as described by the author too, as well as a lot of aches and pains from obesity.

Desperate to regain the control sugar had usurped for years, I knew I had to pay attention to this book. For me, this would include taking note of what I was feeling in addition to what I was eating. Although my emotions had fueled my out-of-control eating many times (I could ruin a diet in less time than it takes people to switch car insurance companies), being aware of my feelings after I ate was key to reining in my food choices and finding the real me.

I chose to blog on the WW online site. I found a creative outlet in playing with words and thoughts instead of eating between meals. I learned to love the sweetness of a comment on my writing more than the fleeting sweetness of a donut. I learned to think beyond the sweetness of sugar to the sweetness of "donut feel good to be able to leave that stuff alone?"

In documenting my feelings, I was able to see how sugar wreaked havoc with my impulse controls and my mental clarity. As I dug deeper and explored the heart of the problem, I could see how sugar robbed me of being my authentic self. Healthier eating became much more attractive. I gained an awareness of the dangers of sugar, and as a bonus, I lost my excess weight as a side effect of my paradigm shift. (Well, it was more like a pair of dimes and a nickel shift, because my first copy of *Potatoes Not Prozac* cost me a quarter at a used book sale.)

My ongoing conclusion about sugar addiction is a matter of awareness. Not everyone is sensitive to sugar, but for anyone who identifies with this, I say pay attention to your body. Notice how you're feeling. (It's part of the gift of being present!) Find what works for a healthy you, and do it with gratitude and without apology. It's a highly customized journey for every individual. It's not a diet; it's a *do* it. It's possible. I'm possible. And you are too!

FROM ZERO TO FIFTY IN POEMS AND PROSE

A Brief Autobiography of My First Fifty Years

As far as my history goes
It's not a great myst'ry for prose
I've had a sweet tooth
Right from my youth
And that's how my story grows.

When I was a child, I used to get my allowance and ride my bike to the store for ten Munch bars. At ten cents each and no sales tax, that's where my buck stopped. I'd hop back on my bike and eat the candy on the way home. A mile and a half per ten candy bars. I don't think I ever considered the fuel economy on that.

Sometimes I had enough extra cash to buy a big bag of M&M's. I'd eat them by myself. If I didn't have money to spend, I would cook fudge frosting for an after-school treat. I experimented with cornstarch and hot cocoa mix and came up with my own microwave instant pudding cups. Mom's brownies were not safe in the freezer when I discovered they were just as good, if not better, frozen as they were thawed. I never considered that she might be saving them for company.

I think these and other incidents with sugar were what triggered my suspicions that my sweet tooth might be a deeper, darker issue. I wondered if it might be akin to alcoholism when I got to that unit in seventh-grade health class. When I substituted the word *candy* for *alcohol* in the diagnostic test for alcoholism, it pretty much described me. I don't know if I talked to anyone about it at the time, but there was a certain shame and fear that I remember. I didn't know what to do about it, though. I didn't feel comfortable discussing it with anyone either.

When I went away to college (I chose to go to my mother's alma mater clear across the country), I encountered all-you-can-eat dorm food. I gained quite a bit of weight using food (as other people might use drugs) to deal with homesickness and other things I didn't know how to deal with. Sweets were escape mechanisms. And even though they were not effective, I still used them. I didn't last long at that school. I returned home, helped take care of my elderly grandfather, and eventually got a job in Boston. I remember getting out of work, racing to a candy shop to get a quarter pound of rocky road fudge, and eating it on the train ride home.

Before I started dating my husband, he offered to help me move from my parents' home in Massachusetts to my new college in Connecticut. I wasn't aware of his romantic interest. I just thought he was being nice. He borrowed a truck from his work, and we went to my folks' house together. He loaded my stuff in the back of the truck, and we were on the way to my new apartment. Several miles down the road, he stopped to check the load. He tested the ropes and determined the load was still secure and safe. Later, probably after we were married, he was reminiscing about that moving experience. I had been sitting as close to the passenger's door as possible. But he was wishing I'd sit a little closer to him. He had considered asking me to move closer to him to keep the load balanced but decided against it. I told him it was just as well he didn't say it. Even though I wasn't overweight at the time, I was sensitive enough about my weight that I might have abandoned ship (or truck) and any possible relationship with him.

When I worked in an office setting, I would bake and bring in cinnamon rolls and other sweets for my coworkers. I baked treats and sweets for my family. And I ate them too. Cookies didn't keep long in my kitchen. If there were leftovers of desserts, I cleaned them up by eating them. Not because I really wanted them, but because I felt compelled to eat them. I was a pro at finding bargains on candy and other sugar-laden confections. I would repeatedly gain weight and then try to lose it.

For all three of my pregnancies, I used my "condition" as a free pass for eating. I didn't drink coffee, but I ate enough for two six-foot men and gained sixty to seventy pounds each time. I lost some of the weight after my babies were born. Sometimes I lost all of the excess weight. But I always gained more back.

I joined Weight Watchers (now known as WW) many times. I participated at the meetings. I was on the bandwagon. I reached goal and achieved lifetime status. And I continually proved my ability to gain weight fast with food-in-control eating. I knew firsthand what Bill Bryson was talking about in *The Lost Continent* when he described Midwestern women gaining weight "all of a sudden and without much notice, like a self-inflating raft from which the pin has been yanked."

I used to go to Jazzercise classes and then stop at a store for a box of cookies. Not to eat just one, but to eat the whole package (well, not the packaging, just the cookies). And candy bars. Milky Way Simply Caramel? Sugar rush. And for what? An empty wallet. A fuzzy feeling in my head. Too-tight clothing. And a craving for more.

I'll say it was a craving for Maureen (the real me) that helped me when I read *Potatoes Not Prozac* by Kathleen DesMaisons. I read the descriptions in the charts and recognized myself. Except it wasn't me. It was someone under the influence of sugar with impaired impulse control, feelings of depression, and basically out-of-control behavior.

I had wondered about sugar for years, and here was some validation in a book with science and facts. It took me a few weeks to actually do something with the information, but I finally got traction to go forward with action. It came to me in rhyme, and it certainly came in time.

I wasn't a youth
That was the truth
I was quickly approaching fifty.
My purpose was simple
Change habit (not wimple)
To be in control would be nifty.

The difference was not in surroundings.
I'd learned I couldn't change that.
The difference had to come from within
And then I could step up to bat.

The book I read clearly defined
What was happening inside my head
Showed me a plan that could help bridge a span
That would help me to eat without dread.

The dread of not having the power to stop
The dread of dressing to have a seam pop.
The dread of not doing things of all kind
Because I was sitting on my big behind.

Focused on what I could cram down my throat
Not really enjoying that big ice cream float.
Trying on clothes in X's size large
Not in a canoe, 'cause I needed a barge.

With the information in *Potatoes Not Prozac*, I had hope for change. I had hope for a better future. I had hope for *me*.

I used some of the simple guidelines I found in *Potatoes Not Prozac*. It describes seven steps for managing sugar sensitivity. The website, which can be found at http://radiantrecovery.com/7-steps/, lists them as follows:

- Eat breakfast with protein.
- Journal what you eat and how you feel.
- Eat three meals a day with protein and a complex carb.
- Take the recommended vitamins and have a potato before bed.
- Shift from white foods to brown foods.
- Reduce or eliminate sugars.
- Create a new life.

Sugar messes with my brain.
It's not the easiest to explain.
There's science and data and all kinds of facts
But the proof that helps *me* is how I acts.

Potatoes Not Prozac does not recommend reducing sugar cold turkey. But I was so convinced that this was my answer, I used my rite of passage into the fifties (colonoscopy) to start with a clean slate just before Thanksgiving 2011. I was amused by the cold-turkey association. I think it helped me get through the test prep and the severe headaches I suffered because I wasn't having any sugar. I went through a couple of days of intense craving, but the clean-slate approach and the hope I had of feeling better got me through to Thanksgiving Day. The painful memory of detox served me well and helped me stay away from sugar on a day where sugar is abundant in pies and pickles and more. But it wasn't in Maureen, and I was thankful.

I do not pretend to understand the science and data involved with sugar addiction. My book is purely anecdotal in nature. I've proven what works for me, and I've had my eyes wide open—no double-blind studies here. I do not suggest that exactly what I did will produce expected results in someone else. If I can help someone start her own search for what works for her, that's great. But the answer is not one size fits all.

I think there *can* be a personal tool kit and plan for anyone to be the healthiest possible for her. For me, it started with awareness that led me to beware of sugar. That, in turn, helped me to care and dare to change my paradigm.

What follows is taken from the blog where I logged my thoughts as I learned to navigate through life with sugar addition. My style is stream-of-conscious thought and sometimes poems—well, quite a lot.

It's one thing to write a blog. But it's a completely different thing to write a book. I had hundreds of thousands of words in hundreds of blog entries. Because I'd shrunk my body by paying attention to how I was feeling, I approached my manuscript in a similar fashion. I wanted to end up with a book I would enjoy reading, but I also wanted my book to be something anyone could enjoy reading. I've been through this manuscript more times than I can count. I've sliced and diced and chopped material. I've repackaged the story that I want to read and share. The rest I canned. Perhaps I'll serve *that* in my next book.

STARTING TO BLOG AND AWAY IT GOES

Gaining Momentum and Losing Weight

In January 2012, I started recording my feelings in a WW blog as part of my quest to control my sugar sensitivity. I remember having several parties to attend. Parties meant lots of food decisions. Here's a peek into how I felt about a day that had two parties:

ONE PARTY DOWN, ONE TO GO
January 14, 2012

I'm super tired from the first party, but I'm not wondering what I can eat. The cake was lovely, and by all reports, delicious. But because I didn't want what goes along with the sugar, I didn't eat the cake. I'll hope for the same resolve this evening. But in the meantime, I need to have another glass of water and get back to cleaning up!

A few days later, I was writing about my prior experience with weight loss:

A FEW POINTS IN RHYME
January 17, 2012

I can't despise the times I've tried
To lose weight in the past.
Having some diet successes
That didn't really last.

I've found a way to look ahead
And to myself be true.
The past is in its place
And I know what *not* to do!

This time I've found
It's not about a diet.

I'm using tools to track what I do
And I'm really glad I tried it.

(This time is less
About the food
But more of how I'm feeling
And just what is my mood.)

Days are much sweeter
Without sugar on my plate
Or snacking all the time—
For meals, I'm glad to wait!

Three cheers for online WW
And what I've learned in a book—
Potatoes Not Prozac has helped a lot—
Sugar addicts! Take a look!

In the process of reading blogs and writing comments, I had some food for thought that sometimes sparked a blog post. The subject of cheating came up fairly often.

WHAT DOES CHEATING MEAN?
January 20, 2012

I felt sad when I read that someone considered it cheating to have a McChicken on her first day with WW. Who was she cheating? Why was it cheating? I guess she felt like she shouldn't have that. I've been there and done that.

So, what's the difference this time? I greatly reduced my sugar intake before I started using WW online to track food and log my feelings and thoughts. If I were to have some sugar right now, I suppose it could be called cheating, but I happen to know it would be cheating *me*, and I'm not interested. I know it cheats me out of feeling good, feeling in control, and feeling like I can.

The WW program is famous for not limiting food choice. There's no need to feel deprived. I know that if I chose to have a hot fudge sundae, I could account for it and still be within the program guidelines. I could have a McChicken sandwich and consider it reasonable for lunch. I don't have to ever be upset with WW for making me feel like I can't eat something. The reason I don't eat certain things is because I know how they make me feel, and I don't want to feel that way.

If I wanted to be upset, I could be upset that my body doesn't tolerate sugar well. I could be upset that I need to be super careful to corral my eating into definite mealtimes. But why be upset when I feel so much better? Why be upset when I feel so liberated from the awful feelings of having food control me? Not everyone is sensitive to sugar. But I am. And I feel best when I embrace the knowledge of what works for me and work it!

Every week on the WW site where I tracked my food and blogged, the weight recording reminder would pop up and I would weigh myself. Because I was following the WW points system as I recorded my foods, I was eating enough to lose weight. And I did lose weight. My weigh-in day was Monday.

MONDAY MORNING BLUES
January 23, 2012

Well, some weight just up and left me
Just four-tenths of a pound.
It may not seem an awful lot,
But I'm glad it's not around.

I struggled with the scale this week
It got inside my head
And I fretted and I fussed a bit
Before I went to bed.

My weight loss is a side effect
Of changing a lifelong habit.
Now I leave the sugar alone.
Before, I used to grab it.

The title's about what I'm wearing.
No, I'm not singing the blues.
Although it's not much, I count it a win
And I'm really quite happy to lose!

I took to blogging like a fish takes to water—or something like that. I was drinking a lot of water instead of eating between meals. I was also writing blog posts between meals when the urge to eat was strong. Sometimes I'd write a little blurb, and sometimes I'd just read and comment on other bloggers' posts. It was a good distraction from my habit of eating for any reason at all. And there was this excitement brewing that I might not stay blobby as I worked my plan.

FROM BLOB TO BLOG
January 23, 2012

I'm writing way too many posts,
Or at least it seems that way.
But while I'm typing out my thoughts
I'm not eating through the day.

It seems to be quite helpful
To read what others say
And make a little comment:
To shout hip, hip, hooray!

If typing were an exercise,
Would it really pay?
Well, my fingers are getting skinny
And it keeps the food at bay!

I remember reading and thinking about control issues. It's a deep subject and hard to understand. This little rhyme was for a time when I thought about myself. What was I doing as I was having less and less control, or responsibility, for my kids as they were leaving the nest? I think I found out that I really needed to take care of me. Although I wasn't writing about my spiritual side, I was finding more balance there too.

IT WORKS FOR ME
January 26, 2012

It works for me.
That's what she said
As she took on her big boss role
The one in charge and the go-to "man"
The one who has control.

It has been said we mothers
Have a need to supervise
To tend to family business
To feed and to advise.

What happens, though, when the children grow
And start to leave the nest?
Sometimes mom's still mom-ing
And thinking she knows best.

That might be absolutely true
But it's usually wise to be quiet
And turn instead to supervise
Her own life and daily diet!

Diet in this case really means
A plan to live each day
To put some weight behind the words
She might be inclined to say.

Of course the optimal life would be
That this happened all along
But some of us might have lost control
And felt like things went wrong.

The point of this poem, I really think,
Is how to have control.
WW helps my body
Prayer helps my spirit and soul.

As I kept up with my tracking and blogging, I found that phrases would trigger thoughts that would help me think about what I was doing. I suppose the process was really a type of therapy. It helped me see inside my head for clues about what and why I was doing things.

THIS IS THE DAWNING OF THE AGE OF ... AWARENESS!
January 30, 2012

I had a not-so-exciting weigh-in last week, but I was aware that numbers don't always show up (or down!) for weigh-in morning. I think awareness is a big deal for me. Being aware of how food affects me has helped me be in control of it. I am very careful around sugar, because I am aware that I have tendencies to let it control me if I eat it in an uncontrolled way. I don't eat between meals, because I am aware that I need a start and stop time to eating so I don't graze my way into being a cow again. (Nothing wrong with cows. It's just that I am *not* one, so I don't want to look like one!) I am aware that sights and smells can be satisfying, and I don't have to eat something to enjoy it. I am aware that my clothes are fitting better. I can, *ah, wear* things that used to be too tight!

One week I started punning the days. And with a little reflection, I decided it was a good exercise. They're not weak days; they're strong days! And the little lessons I learned from the plays on words were a guide!

WHENSDAY IS HERE!
February 1, 2012

Ah yes, a little punning
Won't do any harm.
It's part of how my brain works.
Some think it has some charm.

Others start their groaning
Oh no! A pun! That's bad!
And I just think—I said it first.
They prob'ly wish they had!

The Whensday post was about the day when I would do something. Thursday sounded like taking care of hydration!

THIRSTY THURSDAY
February 2, 2012

Well, I got my fluids in today. I drank lots and lots of seltzer. I shopped at a different grocery store while I was out and found some green apple and vanilla seltzer. Some people don't like seltzer, but I find that it has a filling feeling that helps chase away imagined thoughts of hunger.

By Saturday, I was on a roll.

SATURDAY AWAY
February 4, 2012

I do not want it to be said,
"She sat her day away."
And so I'll get up off my chair
And do some work and play.

Diet mode makes the scale a point of success or failure. But in my mode of managing my sugar addiction, the scale was serving as a snapshot in time. I don't know if I had completely convinced myself of that, but this record of my thoughts shows that I was working on it.

WAIT! WEIGHT! DO TELL ME!
February 13, 2012

What's the point of not knowing? I weighed myself this morning—first thing. I made a decision not to enter it in, though. That could be considered treading in dangerous waters—playing games with the tools instead of using them and trusting them. Kind of goes along with scraping every last bit of yogurt from the measuring cup or shaking crumbs from a napkin into my mouth. But I'm not doing that. And I don't want to do that.

The number I saw this morning was the exact same number I saw last week on Monday morning weigh-in. And that number bumped up the very next day. I wrote a blog post about it and thought I had myself convinced that I would be okay with exactly what happened. Staying the same. I was actually thinking I'd be okay with a gain of miniscule amount.

But I found out otherwise. I wanted a loss. Even two-tenths of a pound. I decided to go for a walk/run on the treadmill and weigh myself again. Short story: I lost 1.2 pounds.

I'd be mentally screaming, "Cheater!" in my head right now if the scale had also registered a higher body fat percentage. But it didn't. I'm going down in body fat. That tells me I'm doing this right. And if by exercising before weigh-in I develop a habit to walk or run for twenty-five minutes before breakfast, I think I win there too!

I'm not going to have the opportunity to weigh myself a lot this week. I'll be away from the scale. I'll see what happens next Monday morning. And report back. Am I fooling myself? I don't think so.

The fact that I wrote another post for my blog in the same day tells me that this weight thing had the potential to weigh me down. Here I am in self-analysis mode shrinking my mind yet again.

DANGEROUS GROUND
February 13, 2012

When I reduced my sugar intake and started losing weight in November 2011, I wasn't at my highest weight ever, but I was headed there—or maybe even higher, based on history. I've lost around thirty pounds since then—a little more than seventeen since the beginning of January.

Because I'm fairly tall and because I dress to minimize my size, people have just started to notice that I've lost weight. It's nice to have the recognition. But it's also scary.

I have to realize I still have more than fifty pounds to lose. And if I tell people that, there is a good possibility they'll say I don't have to. I don't want to hear that. I don't want to believe that. I have to have a grip on the reality that I could lose seventy-five more pounds and still be in a normal weight range for my height. Reality right now is I'm still obese. Not just overweight—obese!

I lost a lot of weight a few years ago. I could actually wear some size-six clothes. I felt good. I became a lifetime member at WW. And I heard someone say, "So what are you going to do now, gain it all back? You look too skinny." I did. I didn't look too skinny. I gained all the weight back. And more. It wasn't that unfiltered person's fault. I did it myself by listening to the wrong signals. I fed my hurt feelings with sugar. And slowly, sometimes quickly, I piled on the weight again.

I could say I'm a different person this time, but I think it's more like I am the same person, I just got rid of some baggage—sugar—and now I'm getting rid of the weight. Pounding it away—using the tracking tools from WW. Yes, I'm *using* the tracking tools along with the guidelines for managing my sugar sensitivity!

One of the biggest concerns for me was sustainability of my program. I knew I needed to be able to stay in control wherever I was. I was pleased to get through a ski trip and feel successful with my plan.

SUCCESS!
February 20, 2012

I was a bit nervous about last week's ski trip. Typically, I eat way too much when I go skiing. And typically, I gain weight. But this time was different. I had a plan. I had my tracking tools. And I worked them. The best plans and the best tools don't work unless they're worked!

I enjoy skiing. Even at my highest weight, I enjoyed it. There was something about the ease of moving down the slopes that made me feel light as a feather. And it wasn't my down jacket. I've enjoyed skiing even more this year. I'm not at my lightest weight. (I'm still considered obese by the BMI calculator.) But I've been using my plan and the tools, and I am confident they work when I use them. As far as the skiing goes, I've had some lessons on how to use my skis (tools) more effectively, and the confidence that has given me has increased my enjoyment of the sport.

Several years ago, I took a spill on an expert trail called Spillway. It's an aptly named trail! The problem I had was mostly psychological. I got to a part of the trail where I couldn't see my way down. When I went over the knoll, I panicked, lost confidence, and fell. Out of control. I wanted to walk the rest of the way. But it was too steep. Somehow, I made it to the bottom, but that was it for Spillway. I felt defeated by that trail.

I had been back to that mountain several times, but I hadn't attempted Spillway again. Some years it was because the trail was closed. And other years it was because when we went over the trail on the lift, we could hear the skiers and snowboarders scraping ice all the way down. This year was different. This year we had packed powder with three inches of fresh powder on top.

Spillway is still a black diamond, and it still has a section where you just can't see where the trail goes, but I had confidence in my tools and my ability to use them. And I did it! Several times! I didn't fall at all. My turns were linked. I didn't snowplow! It was a challenge, for sure, but I did it and enjoyed it!

I still have some challenges to overcome with skiing. I attempted a trail that I wasn't ready for. I got to the bottom (some of it by hiking and carrying my skis), but it really was more than I could handle (trees and rocks and steep). I need some more lessons and perhaps better equipment and fitness level before I would even consider it again.

I'm seeing a parallel here. And it has to do with my weight-loss journey. Last year, I got some lessons from *Potatoes Not Prozac*. I learned about how to manage my sugar addiction. WW tracking tools help me apply the lessons. I like to think of it as basic reading (blogs), writing (blogs and comments), and arithmetic (adding up food and activity points and subtracting pounds).

I've tried the weight-loss trail many times. And a few times I've gotten down. But most of the time I've taken a spill. And all of the times I've ended up feeling defeated because I gained the weight back.

This time, though, I have some confidence (I'm sure it's because I've greatly limited my sugar intake), because I have good tools and good instructions. I'm able to use them effectively. Yes, I'm still obese. But

I'm only 6.2 pounds away from simply overweight! And from there, it's looking very doable to get to an ideal, healthy, weight for me.

As I logged my food and blogged my moods, my brain played with word sounds and rhymes. Sometimes I would notice the puns as I wrote them, and other times, I'd find them as I read over what I'd just written.

HERTZ (SO BAD)
February 27, 2012

I find this blog is an outlet
For my creative spark.
It gives my brain some exercise
And sheds light on the dark!

I'm finding it quite helpful
To write what I've done and why.
Being aware of what's going on
Is making me do more than try.

This time on plan, I'm quite active:
I'm using the tools with success.
It's not a matter of, "Maybe I will,
Or I think I'll try, I guess."

This time I'm blogging, I'm logging, I'm jogging
(Mostly my mind but soon with my feet).
I've no need to count out extra food points.
I'm typing, not wond'ring what I can eat!

As I lost weight and inches, I had clothes to measure myself by. Some of the clothes were hand-me-ups from my daughters. I had hopes of fitting into them, and this was a day those hopes were reality.

A LITTLE OVER THE TOP. BUT I'M NOT EATING.
February 28, 2012

I'm wearing my daughter's hand-me-up shirt—
It's a J.Crew trim-fitted large
I've had for quite a while
But it didn't fit on my barge.

As I steadily worked my collection of tools
And my poundage started to drop,
I would try this shirt as a measurement
But the buttons still wanted to pop.

My arms barely fit in the long thin-striped sleeves
They looked like sausages—wurst!
Forget about wearing unbuttoned, untucked
If I tried, I would look like I'd burst!

I've continued to work the WW tools
Blogging with vigor and vim!
And this morning, with ease, my arms slipped through those sleeves
I buttoned completely and then tucked it in!

Not only did I have a creative outlet with words, but I was also creative with food. This meal was fun to make, fun to write about, and fun to eat. I suppose it was also fun to track with all the healthy vegetables in it.

BREAKFAST ABROAD, RiGHT AT HOME!
March 1, 2012

My breakfast this morning was Seoul food
Made in Morean style.
My friend from Korea cooks this way
I'd not had such food for a while.

I started out with a frying pan
A teaspoon of sesame oil.
Set the burner at medium heat—
I didn't want it to boil.

I sliced up half an onion
(the brand, it was OSO sweet)
And then I thought of more veggies
That would make my breakfast a treat!

Mushrooms, sliced fresh
A cup full, I guess(h)
Red pepper, diced, a cabbage leaf, sliced
Basmati rice (not Korean, but nice).

A handful of spinach, I thought to put in it(ch)
A clove of garlic and more:
Soy sauce, a tablespoon, a sprinkle of ginger,
An egg (not poached) bought at the store.

I added a single carrot,
Nicely julienned.
(I used this technique mostly
For how it would sound when I penned!)

Yes, as I cooked my breakfast,
This poem was starting to form.
I really had a lot of fun
While I was cooking up this storm.

I not only had fun while I fixed it,
I enjoyed eating this bibimbap.
And now that I've written and posted this poem
I think I'll go for a … wok.

I think I was a little concerned about the rhyming here. But I worked it through and got a smile out of it. It helped that I knew it was someone's birthday!

MY EXCUSE AND A LITTLE MORE
March 2, 2012

There are times in my life that I wonder
If, really, I might just be sick.
I start to say something, my brain starts to race
For the next rhyming word it should pick.

For a while it is fun
Then the novelty's done
To speak normal I must pause.
Then after some time, I can talk without rhyme
I really don't know the cause.

Well, after some thought
(Valid, or not)
I think that I've found an excuse.
In my formative years and those of my kids
I was read to, and read, Dr. Seuss!

Happy birthday, Dr. Seuss!
No, thanks, I don't want some cake.
I'm a Weight Watcher now, and that stuff is allowed
But I know what I can and can't take!

*My blog title (Pointing the Way) was word play on the points system of
WW. Sometimes I'd work "points" into my posts.*

THE POINT OF NO RETURN
March 2, 2012

I enjoy words. Reading them and writing them. Some of my posts might
make a person think I need to go see a shrink, but this blog is helping me
with that! Seriously. I think blogging works as therapy that helps with
the psychological part of "waist management"!

I also enjoy food. I would say too much enjoyment of food is what got
me to needing to lose weight, but I don't think that is a true statement.
When I think of all the food I ate just to eat—just on an impulse, just
for comfort, just out of boredom—I know I didn't become obese by
enjoying food.

I think I enjoy food now. I know I appreciate it more. I understand how
it affects me. I know if I should just enjoy the sight and smell of it or
actually eat it. That doesn't prevent me from my enjoyment of preparing
food. While I've been blogging this morning, I've made an *apearantly*
apple pie (pear and apple) and cinnamon rolls. I won't eat them. They
are for people who can handle them.

Recently I read a blog that talked about empty points. And that's where
I came up with my title. There are some foods that just don't give much
return for their point value.

On my previous attempts to be a Weight Watcher, I think my downfall
usually began with using my points on junk. Maybe I'd have several
Smart Ones desserts at a time. I would justify them because they had the
WW logo on them along with the tracking values. I figured they were
just fine as long as I counted them! And then supper (and sometimes
lunch) would have to be vegetables and water if I wanted to stay on
program with my allotted points. Sometimes I would just eat vegetables.
But eventually, I would quit and gain weight. (And that was a pattern I
started to hate!)

I can enjoy food more now that I understand what it can do to me. I have memories of wonderful tastes. And the sights and smells are enough for me. If I had one bite, the experience would be just for a few moments, and that too would become a memory. But then I'd have to deal with the consequences of sugar in my brain, which would lead to trouble with controlling my impulses. (I have decades of proof for that one.) And I'd be in danger of gaining back everything I've already lost.

Eating junk food, for me, is like a point of no return. Falling off the wagon. Oh, I think I'd be able to get back on the wagon again even though it's hard. I know I'll have to be careful for the rest of my life. But I'm enjoying the ride on the wagon. Why bother falling off?

I saw March fourth as a day of action, and this is how I handled it.

SUNDAY
March 4, 2012

I was glad for a good day today. There was a lot of natural food available, but that wasn't the focus. And I am thankful. "Let your soul delight itself in fatness" is a good kind of fatness, and I don't want to lose sight of that!

My body isn't delighting in fatness. (If it were, I'd be de-lighting— gaining weight.) Weigh-in is tomorrow. There is a slim chance that this body will break out of the realm of obesity and join the ranks of the simply overweight.

Tomorrow is a new day! I have the option to make it a good one. I know I'll need help along the way. And I know where to get it.

I didn't get out of the ranks of obese the next day, but I managed to keep my spirits up!

HELLO, SCALE! IT'S GOOD TO SEE YOU!
March 5, 2012

Down two point four
Had it been just one more
I'd have been out of the ranks of obese.
But it's okay to wait
I'll just watch o'er my plate
And stay far from things cooked in hot grease!
(Well, I don't tend to eat fried food anyway. But it rhymed!)

I was thinking about my appointment with the scale on Monday mornings. I actually weigh myself through the week, so I'm not usually very surprised by the official weigh-in. What I'm learning is that my weight fluctuates a few pounds up and down. But the general trend is down. Because I'm using my tools. With purpose. And on purpose.

Although the scale number doesn't always have the number I think I'd like to see on weigh-in morning, it has the number of how many pounds I weigh at that given moment! I've recommended googling an article, "Why the scale lies." But it doesn't really lie. It *can* provide cause for self-searching, though.

My number this morning is actually a pound heavier than I saw on one of my unofficial weight checks last week. I had been excited about the possibility of being officially just overweight and not obese. But even if I were there, I still wouldn't be at my goal. I'm not done with the plan. And when I'm at goal, I still won't be done with the plan. This is a lifetime thing, and I'm not going to pout about the timing (today).

So back to my weigh-in this morning. It was a good one. I really shouldn't be losing over two pounds a week—for the health of it. I had a good week. I happened to eat ham at two meals yesterday. I didn't get official activity for two days. I could have had more water to drink. But I'm not beating myself up.

Here's to a new week. And, well, maybe not quite like the excitement and anticipation of seeing a good friend again, but I think I just might look forward to stepping on the scale next Monday morning!

I googled WW codes and jargon one day and got a key to make sense of what I was reading in other blogs. I had lots of ideas for the letters I was seeing, but the posts made much more sense when I knew what the writer had intended!

LSV-NSV'S
March 7, 2012

Large-scale victory. Non-scale victories. I weighed myself this morning, and I'm unofficially simply overweight. I'm not obese! And it's not just by a tenth of a pound! I'll wait until my official weigh-in on Monday to actually count it, but to me, this is a large-scale victory! I also have several non-scale victories to note. I actually think they have a bit of magnitude, so I'm not quite sure they should be called non-scale.

This week, I have exercised for twenty minutes on the treadmill before I blogged. That's been three days in a row. Usually when I think I have something to write, I want to do it right *now*. (This reminds me a bit of when I lacked control over eating!) I've decided it's a good exercise for me to wait on the blog post. I allow myself to jot an idea down on a piece of paper, but I don't indulge in full-scale blogging.

I'm getting exercise at the beginning of the day, because even though after just about every post I think I probably won't think of more ideas, I seem to always find something to write about! And just as an aside, I find it slightly funny that I can be more focused on what I want to write than what I want to eat!

I took our new skis to the ski shop for binding release checks. Big deal one: although I am still above goal, I didn't feel like I had to whisper my weight or write it on a piece of paper for the techie. Big deal two: my current ski boots are designed for large calves. (I used to look like a small herd!) But the last time I used them, I noticed they felt a bit big— not in length, but in girth. So, today, I tried on a pair of boots we got on clearance for less than twenty dollars a few years ago (too good of a deal to leave at the store).

They are high-tech ski boots, and I couldn't even get my foot in when we bought them. But today, I could get my foot in and buckle them. Today, they felt good! And today, the guy at the ski shop thought I should go with them, because they were a superior boot. He said the other boots (I brought both pairs) were really designed to hold watermelons!

There's a concept in weight loss that is dreaded. It's a stall that folks call a plateau. I hadn't reached that stage, but I had read about it. This is how I processed it in my head.

ODE TO A PLATE (PLATEAUED)
March 8, 2012

My brain was convoluting words
As it often will.
And thoughts began to swirl around
Weight losses close to nil.

Since joining for this final time
(I have to believe that's so)
I've steadily gone down in numbers

And not hit the dreaded plateau.

I've done this plenty of times in my life
And read quite a number of blogs
To know that this thing about weight loss
Is not always like falling off logs.

There are numerous theories of what to do
In this dreadful and frightening stage.
I've proven one thing to *not* work:
To quit and stomp off in a rage.

That, in itself, might earn extra points.
But, often, the ensuing binge
Would crash my wagon and loosen my doors
So they'd come right off at the hinge.

The answer I'm reading
Quite a bit of late
Is perhaps there is not
Enough food on your plate!

While this rhyme's form (or lack thereof)
Is not anything like an ode
To start losing more weight
Fill up your plate
With what it really is owed!

Originally, my thought was to blog about my moods. But I realized my moods came through no matter what I wrote about. I suppose I could call it the write way for me to use the blogging tool! The next few posts were a run of points. I remember googling phrases that included the word point and then thinking of ways to write about them for my situation.

OFFENSiVE POiNTS
March 14, 2012

Early on in my blogging experience, I wrote a post about pointed remarks. In a previous WW experience, I had taken offense at something someone had said and let it derail me in my weight-management efforts.

Last night we were talking about what it means to take offense. And in thinking about it, I realized I do not need to take offense at anything someone says to me if I am secure in who and what I am. The speaker who would be offensive may or may not intend the offense. It may be a point of ignorance or insensitivity or pure malice. But it belongs to that person, and I do not need, or want, to take it on myself.

Sugar affects my brain and body in a way that interferes with all good intentions regarding reasonable eating. I think I can call it offensive, but I choose to not be offended by it. I don't take it in without protein as a buffer in the digestive or metabolic process.

I find it helpful to remember what I was thinking about when I was writing. Some things are easier to picture than others.

SNAPPING POINT
March 15, 2012

The idea for this post came when I was looking at some pictures from 2004. I remember how much I weighed (about twenty pounds less than I do right now). And I remember thinking when I printed the pictures that I looked fat in those snapshots.

I have shied away from most cameras in the past few years. But there have been a few occasions (my son's wedding, for one) when I couldn't avoid having my picture snapped. I try for the winning smile—who could focus on anything else? But when I see the results, I'm not fooled. It's flabulous, not fabulous. It's highly likely that I'm the only one who assesses a picture of me like that, the emphasis being on me. I don't often see the excess weight on other people—in pictures or in person.

Another thing for me to consider on these unavoidable planned picture occasions is that I've usually dieted like mad beforehand. But not mad enough. Or maybe it hadn't been happy enough. And most likely because it was a diet and not a program for life.

Those snapping points have sometimes been the prod to get more serious about weight loss. But it wasn't a quest to look better for a snapshot that changed my picture. It was a quest to be healthy—the picture of health.

There's a certain joy in the realization of change for the better.

BECAUSE I CAN
March 20, 2012

I was driving along today and remembering how I used to drive along with detours through fast-food restaurants and stops at convenience stores. I wondered why I used to stop and buy a "treat" for myself. I wasn't often *really* hungry. But it was something I did. Perhaps it was a few dollars burning a hole in my pocket (and my sugar addiction wanting another hit): "I'll get it because I can!"

Today as I was driving along and came to several former detour points, I happily kept driving. There was some money in my pocket (probably more than there used to be!), but I kept going. Because I can!

Although I took higher-level math in college, I think this is where I really came to terms with it.

INFLECTION POINT
March 26, 2012

This is actually a term in differential calculus. It's the point on a curve where it changes from positive to negative or vice versa (so says Wikipedia, anyway). Inflection also has to do with a change in the pitch or tone of the voice (thank you, Dictionary.com).

So, to quote someone who has commented on my blog and wall, "What's the point?" Well, we're dealing with curves—quite a few curves. And there seem to be a lot of positives to negatives and negatives to positives, negatives that are positives and positives that are negative. It's a wonder that anyone can make sense of this whole thing. But the results—if you can differentiate everything properly—are quite amazing.

Some of us are dealing with voices in our heads. Not so much different personalities or schizophrenia, but perhaps the superego? I'm "aFreud" I'm not too familiar with that branch of psychology, but good-old Wikipedia has a definition that fits. ("The superego plays the critical and moralizing role.")

Anyway, there seems to be a point where a person realizes the negative voices have to change to positive. A little compassion in the tone. Something kinder and gentler (but not beating around the bush—which on The Phrase Finder website means to "prevaricate and avoid coming to the point").

I find it helps me when I read blogs and comments on a regular basis. And I think it is very helpful to write blogs and comments. There's a lot of positive reinforcement and positive encouragement going on. And when I am encouraging others, there's a point where I realize I could take the same approach to my own situation. I think it can be called *inflectious*!

Changing a negative inflection to positive can make weigh-ins be negative, which is really positive. It positively makes a difference! It points to a change in my head and a change in the shape of my curves.

My husband and I used to hike a lot. I remember seeing signs announcing a view, and it usually meant a time to stop and see more than just the trail. I found it helpful to do this figuratively from time to time. It was nice that my figure was shrinking too!

VISTA POINT
April 2, 2012

I've been chugging along on this journey, and it's time to stop and take a look. No, I'm not stopping the journey, but just taking a step outside of myself for a reality check. The fog from sugar has been gone since November. I've been faithfully tracking my foods and moods with the WW eTools since January.

As of this morning, I've lost fifty pounds since my highest high. I haven't set my healthy weight yet, but losing another fifty pounds would put me midrange for my height and bone size. There have been a few moments lately when I realized I was at a weight that I didn't really think I'd ever get to again (as in that low). And then I think about being this weight before.

When we were headed to a family reunion in Florida in 2000, I was horrified that I had let myself get so heavy. I think it was my first time to buy clothes with an X after the number. I had weighed more before that, but I had also been pregnant at the time. I've yo-yoed around a few times and passed this number, but I was so far above it this time, I really think I had figured on never coming back through. I want to remember this as I keep losing weight. It's possible!

Minus fifty pounds, the real me is starting to show. I look way better than I looked a few months ago. I'm not wearing clothes that are too tight (how it was when I started), and I'm not wearing clothes that are too loose. I'm wearing clothes that fit. I'm getting compliments. My first thought is: "But I have another fifty pounds to lose." And then I have to look at where I was and where I am now and say, "Thank you for noticing!"

Because I'm fairly tall, I can carry around a lot more weight than my shorter friends. But I don't want to just give the illusion of being at a healthy weight. I really want it to be so. I don't want to hide excess pounds. Even if they can't be seen, I don't want them!

Yesterday someone commented on my weight loss. She asked me if I was getting ready for my big birthday (fifty). I said no. I was getting ready for the rest of my life! And it felt good to say that and mean it!

So here at this vista point, I see some realities. I used to be obese, but now I'm overweight. I'm starting to look better. There's a healthy weight I can reach, and I'm headed there. I'm doing this.

I'd see or think of a phrase, and my mind would twist it to fit my blog. This concept of point-blank has helped me several times.

POINT-BLANK
April 3, 2012

This is not an empty post. It's a thought about targets. Targets so close, I can hit them dead-on. (And I'm not talking about being first in line on sale day at the store!) It's about point-blank shooting: no change from the aim to the goal.

I could get overly concerned about my long-range goal to live at a healthy weight. It's about fifty pounds away. Yes, that thought could make me a little shaky. But what I'm shooting at point-blank is living toward a healthy goal. That's an everyday thing. Or, point-blank, it's a moment-to-moment thing!

So, point-blank goals: Tracking my food on the WW site and using all of my allotted points. That's a pretty easy one for me. Exercise before blogging. Bull's-eye! Reading and commenting on blogs. On target! The list goes on. And they're all fairly easily achievable. I've been doing them repeatedly since January!

My accuracy and precision are bloggable! The side effect has been steady weight loss! In the process of time and tenacity, I blow through the targets and get closer and closer to the long-range goal. When I'm in point-blank range of that, though, it's probably best not to blow that target apart. But the goal is really to stay in point-blank range.

Some points were more serious than others. But life is like that, and this was me dealing with life. And death.

END POINT
April 5, 2012

A dear friend of mine had been struggling with weight gain. It was possibly from stress eating. She had a lot going on. And then she found out she had cancer. She lost about a hundred pounds in a very short time. She looked good. She had a wonderful spirit about her. She was living with cancer. It wasn't defining her, but it was killing her. She gave it a strong push back. And she's lived way longer than most who are diagnosed with that form of cancer. She has continued to make the most of her time. Living her faith. Loving, caring for, and encouraging everyone around her.

Over the years, she and I had commiserated about the annoyances of needing to lose weight. And when she lost so much so quickly, she joked to me it was a very effective weight-loss method, but not at all recommended.

She noticed I was working on changing some of my eating habits. And she gave me encouragement.

My friend has great faith. She understands that our bodies are only a temporary thing. Our true being goes on when the dust is put aside. There is a sense of joy and sorrow interwoven. And wonderful peace. She's on her deathbed. I will miss her. But I understand her faith and trust and that she is ready to go on.

For me, I'm still enthusiastic about all I'm doing with the WW online tools. But I'm aware there's going to be an end point. I'm glad the goal for my body is not just a number. It's to live healthy, to be thankful, and to embrace the wonderful opportunities and privileges that life holds. And when it is time to leave it behind, I want to be ready to do just that.

My friend passed away on April 8, 2012. Because emotional eating can be such a problem area, I found it helpful to write right through the experience. Eating can seem so shallow at times, and yet, there's an urge to drown in it to avoid the pain of facing reality. I think writing served as a life preserver for me in this case.

TO THE POINT OF TEARS
April 16, 2012

Tears express what we can't in words—
Hearts spilling out through our eyes
Emotions raw from joys or woes
The visual sign of heart sighs.

Response to the tears
Doesn't have to be much
A hug or a smile—
A sympathetic touch.

The greatest poetry
Of all time
Can be in a gesture
Without any rhyme.

This week will end in a memorial service for my friend. Thoughts of her life—what and who she was—will be close by. And there may be some tears. But my purpose is to embrace the experience. To recognize the power and strength behind and in her life. Yes, there will be lots of food. But that is not the focus or the answer or the hiding place for any or all of the feelings that may come.

As I was thinking about tears, I wondered if they are a part of a healing process. And although I don't like to cry, I've been aware sometimes that I just need to. And in a healthy way, it's a wonderful thing when I'm with someone who can respond to that wordless communication with just the right response. Heart to heart.

This topic is hard to express in words
It's been good for me to try.
I'm realizing in a significant way
It's okay to have a good cry.

Food is there for nourishment
For my body—not for my soul.
And when everything is in balance—
That's when I am whole.

As I have worked through my writing, I've been aware of the serious and silly sides of me. I think it's good to have a balance. Perhaps that goes for life in general. And here is some silly!

FASHION POINTS
April 16, 2012

I threw away some tights today
They weren't Parisian style
But more like from southwestern France
They'd been Toulouse awhile!

I've quite a bit of work to do
Revamping my whole closet
Getting rid of things too large
Making a Goodwill deposit.

While I'm at the thrift store,
I'll find some things to wear
Perhaps I'll try some new styles
I've never had nerve to dare!

No, I'll probably stick with the classics
That don't go out or in.
And save my big shopping for goal weight—
My lifetime of being thin!

What fun to venture out shopping
Where to? Some readers might ask.
Prob'ly department store clearance
Or Marshalls or T.J. Maxx!

I've never been a fashion plate
I've used them mostly for food.
Perhaps this rhyme will serve some smiles
And lighten someone's mood.

Weigh-ins could generate nervousness before and excitement or disappointment afterward. I tried to keep the games out of weigh-in days to keep it real. Some of my online friends reported shaving their legs before weigh-in, but the idea of flossing first amused me this day.

SiLLY RHYME
April 30, 2012

Perhaps I will compose a rhyme
About my little loss
That might have been a smidge bigger
Had I waited to weigh-in post-floss.

Actually, it wasn't that small of a drop
If you think about the tenths.
I lost a total of twelve of them
And I'm not looking for where they went(h).

I don't follow the fashion flow
But I'm happy to follow this trend
Of slow and steady down, down, down.
And there, my rhyme is penned.

Yes, it's rather silly
But it's meant in the spirit of fun.
I do what I do—what works for me
For this losing weight thing to be done!

It's not the *done* of finality
Like I won't be using the plan
But the done that goes with doing it
For lifetime—'cause I *can*!

*This post was inspired by an online friend. She posted as her status a
comment about not allowing negative thoughts about self. My comment
to her was: "Picture this: if a negative thought crops up, do not develop it!"*

POiNT AND SHOOT
May 10, 2012

I think puns are funny, but this is serious stuff. Self-criticism can get
out of control. Reality checks are one thing, but self-criticism can be
dangerous. When it gives a skewed view that defies improvement, it's
really bad. If there happen to be surroundings that assist in that kind of
criticism, that's even worse.

Even though I grew up in a very supportive environment, I was usually
able to twist most encouragement around to be critical of me. For myself,

I think the self-criticism in a surrounding of sugar addiction was part of why I didn't stick with a healthy weight when I got there the last time. Maybe it was because only the number was healthy and not the rest of me. Hmmm. That's a weighty thought. And that's what I'm writing about.

I like to think of the scale reading as a snapshot in time. (Point and shoot, if you will.) It's a record of where I am at that given moment. It's not the destination. I'm not staying there. And it's not what defines me.

I'll still do the scale snapshots when I'm at my healthy weight. My goal is to live there.

Some posts of self-reflection turned into a cheering squad.

THE I'DS OF MAY
May 15, 2012

I wrote it in a comment:
Something I would have done
If I'd thought a little better—
If I'd fought a battle and won.

I'd have weighed myself monthly at lifetime
Whether I'd had or not had to pay
And I'd have used the tools effectively
If I'd known what I know today.

Ah yes, beware the I'ds.
It's usually of March, they say.
But here it is—two months hence
There's great hope in the month of May.

I wish I May
I wish I mighter
Do some things
That will make me lighter.

Yes! Indeed I may!
Permission is granted
To get rid of the I'ds
Of which I ranted!

It's time to spring
Right into summer
And not sit and mope
That life is a bummer.

I *may* rise up and *do it*!
There's hope in a changing tide.
For a really good kind of shrinking
And breaking into stride.

I *may* eat the foods I like
And I will track them, every one.
I *may* blog about my thoughts
When my activity points are done.

I *may* eat three good meals a day
And a snack combined with cheese.
I *may* have a baked potato
(With chives and butter, please).

I *may* work the tools
That work for me so well
And then in rhyme, or maybe some prose,
About them I will tell.

I *may* make puns
That are so lame
They *may* need crutches
Or something to blame.

Some weeks from right now
It will be just great
To not moan the I'ds
Cause I *did*! (And lost weight!)

When I was shrinking my book, some blog posts seemed pretty wacky on the surface. But on closer look, they made a lot of sense. It might seem like a wild ride, but it was all about keeping me safe from the sugar monster. I decided to keep this one in.

JUST DONUT
May 23, 2012

I'm fresh off the treadmill. I had a great weigh-in this morning. Down 2.4 pounds since Monday. I guess I'm not full of bologna anymore. I'd say I am on a roll, but I'm thinking donuts this morning.

Donut feel great to be in control of food instead of food-controlled? Donut feel great to sit down at the computer with a tall glass of water and catch up with the online community? (Yes, I did think ketchup, but decided it just donut work tastefully here.)

Actually, I was really thinking of Nike's slogan: *Just Do It.*

Yesterday, I was thinking of changing my weigh-in day from Monday to Wednesday. I had been thinking about it for a while, and I finally got to the point of just doing it. I did seem to need to write a poem about it first, but now I've just donut. And it feels good.

To look at this word from all angles (picture an angular donut?), the gist of *Potatoes Not Prozac* for me was, "Just donut eat sugar carelessly." Paying attention to that (and my body) has helped me get rid of my cravings and impulse eating. I suppose I could call this a lifesaver, but in this case, it's not quite as catchy.

Living with sugar sensitivity is an everyday thing. It doesn't go away when I go away on vacation. It still has to be managed, or it ends up managing me. Here is an account of my first major slip. Or perhaps it was a general one.

GETTYSBURG
May 29, 2012

Generally, I've stayed on program since January 2, 2012. Staying on program, to me, means tracking my food and activity and writing in my blog. They are simple tools of awareness. I use them, and I've lost more than fifty pounds since November. I recorded one little blip up, but that was gone in two days.

This past weekend, my husband and I went on a camping trip with our sixteen-year-old daughter and one of her friends. Another couple had suggested a trip to Gettysburg, and we joined them at the Caledonia State Park just a little west of the famous battlefield town.

I could go into a complete blow-by-blow description of what happened to me and my program, but I'll just compare it to history. Back in 1863, the Rebels were caught off guard. They didn't have good information (they didn't know the size of the enemy they were facing), there was a lack of trust in some of the tools (spy information), they couldn't execute coordinated attacks, and they had overconfidence coming off a recent huge victory. Initial perceived success on the first day of battle just reinforced the overconfidence. By the third day, they were sorely defeated into retreating back home.

I am not a Civil War scholar. But little snippets that I remember from our tours, reading material, and museum experiences seem awfully familiar to me.

On Friday morning, I stepped on the scale and saw a number I hadn't seen since 2004. That was a big confidence booster! We left home a little late but not bad. We stopped for lunch and supper, and I noted what I ate so I could track it when I got home.

I will spare the rest of the details and note that overtiredness, heat, sugar (I ate two cookies on Saturday evening and got into the trail mix on the way home), lack of information (no computer, no blogging community, and the enemy was bigger than I thought), overconfidence from previous victory, poor (or lack of) planning and timing, and poor ground (too much grazing) all contributed to my feeling of defeat (out of control) by the third day.

I have had it with the rebel eating stuff. I may have to endure cravings and headaches today, but I feel like I'm back on good ground. This morning, I have entered in my tracker, as best as I remember, the poor food choices I made over the weekend. I have a deficit on my weeklies that I may or may not be able to make up today. But it's recorded. I'm using my tools again.

I walked for twenty minutes this morning. And I've written this blog entry. I'm going to spend some time reading and commenting on blogs while I do laundry. My tools are with me, and I'm using them. The battles will likely continue, but I'm seeing victory (just not overconfidently). As a whole, it's good.

I learned that battles didn't end automatically with a feeling of normalcy again. This next post woke me up to how fragile I was feeling. For me, using the tools for success meant using all of the tools. Blogging included.

INADEQUATE

May 30, 2012

A Google search produced this definition: "Not adequate; lacking the quality or quantity required; insufficient for a purpose." And that about sums up my feeling for a blog post today.

I weighed myself and chose to wait until after I exercised to do my official weigh-in. I managed to squeak in a no gain, no loss. I've done fine with activity and tracking. But I haven't felt like blogging. I didn't know what to say. But I'm using the tools, and this has worked. And I want it to work still.

In less than a month, we will be going to a family reunion. Family reunions have typically been a frantic time for me to try to lose weight. And that works about as well as a diet. Most of my relatives are super skinny and athletic. And short. Even when I'm at a healthy weight, I look huge next to them. They're all very nice people. Most (if not all) of the problem is in my head.

Maybe that's what I need to write about. It's the next big thing on the schedule. I have to think about it. And plan for it. I won't have access to my regular tools. But I've had a practice run. I can see where I need to pay more attention without being obsessive so I can enjoy the time for what it is. I don't want to let my weight or food define me or my experience. I won't be at my healthy weight for this reunion, but I'll be way closer than I was in January. And I'm planning to be closer than I am today.

Here I am at the end of the post. I have discovered I did have something to write about. And I have reinforced in my mind that blogging helps in some measure. I would also like to note that I just rested my left hand on the corner of the computer table, and I could see airspace between my ring and my ring finger!

I'm not sure what triggered this post, but it doesn't matter. It's a classic example of what can happen in my head sometimes. I took it out for a ride in my blog.

TIME FOR A TUNE-UP?

May 31, 2012

When I was in high school, I was on the college bowl team. One of the questions asked was, "What is needed to do a tune-up for most cars?"

This was back in the seventies, and the correct answer was points, plugs, and a condenser.

Things may have changed since then, but the idea works for a blog post. At least it works for me!

My dad and mom owned an auto repair shop in Boston. When I was a kid, family supper conversations usually included car stories (we had our own live Car Talk every night). Some of the stories were hilarious, and some of them were sad. My dad is a great storyteller, so they were all pretty much interesting. I don't know much about how cars work, but I do have some of the lingo.

How does this tie in with my weight-loss journey? Buckle up!

Oil Changes: This can change everything. Healthy oils—eat them. Whether you cook with them or mix them in your oats for more horsepower, use them. Don't be afraid to eat things with high fat content. I've done well eating avocados and peanut butter. Not together, but I eat (and track) them regularly.

Timing Belt: I have start and stop times for eating. I don't graze between meals. It helps with impulse control. And I've bought a smaller-size belt that I can buckle on the third notch in!

Brakes: An important control feature. Know when and how to stop, whether it's eating or obsessing about how to count something. WW is a set of tools. And this is an important one. Stop. And then go on.

Tires: If I find that I'm worn out, I know I need to change things up a bit. Maybe get some activity points. Or get to bed earlier if I'm exhausted. Both things are helpful in weight loss. And that means less of a spare.

Transmission: Get in gear and communicate through the online community. It should be an automatic go-to when things are rough or when I've fallen into the clutches of bad habits. I've found the standard response is helpful, encouraging, and enlightening (very helpful for weight loss).

Bearings: Know what the tools are and how to use them. Get your bearings and move forward in life and down on the scale.

Fluids: Very important to keep the levels up. From washer fluid, to antifreeze. If the radiator runs dry, there's big trouble. It would drive you to drink. Water you doing to hydrate?

Head Gasket: A big part of the journey is above the neck. It's wise to keep it in good repair. Omega-3 helps me a lot.

Back to the tune-up. Most of my blog posts have **points**, **plugs** for WW and *Potatoes Not Prozac*, and a purpose to **condense**(r) my size. No wonder they help me move forward on this journey!

Car repair issues can be daunting. And weight-loss issues can be too. A good way to deal with both is to be aware and pay attention to signs and signals that something might be wrong. Diagnostic tests, warning lights, hunches, sounds, smells, and feels are all important things to watch. Good maintenance practices can prevent many problems. And if I'd paid more attention, that's where I'd be—maintenance. But I've found a good repair shop. The tools are working. And I'm enjoying the ride again!

Part of my preparation for vacation was to examine possibilities and revisit history. I think it was all to make my story better. Our family reunion was on houseboats at Lake Roosevelt. I'd never done such a thing, but I could think about my possible options.

JUSTIFICATION. JUSTAVACATION.
June 3, 2012

I was thinking about our upcoming vacation and how I need to get my mind around what I'm going to do with my tools while I'm gone. I don't think I'll have a lot of access to the online WW tools. I won't have a lot of say in the menu while we're on the houseboats. But I'm pretty sure there will be enough choices that I'll be okay.

My lessons learned from my Battle of Gettysburger tell me that whatever I eat, I need to have start and stop times to meals—no grazing. I also need to make sure I stay away from most sugars. If I have fruit, I need to have some protein with it. I might decide to just skip the afternoon snack thing if protein is not an option.

This plan doesn't have so much to do with WW as it does with my level of enjoyment during the trip.

I know from experience that when my impulse controls are compromised because of sugar, I focus more on food than what's around me. I don't want to do that. I want to enjoy the people I'm with. I want to enjoy the things we do and the sights we'll see. There may be days when I just cannot track my food. And I'm thinking that is okay. Justification? It's justavacation.

Vacations are a variation from normal day-to-day living. One definition could be taking a break from regular work or routine to relax. There are things a person doesn't (or shouldn't) stop doing just because she's on vacation. Like breathing. Like keeping true in relationships—natural and spiritual.

Many times on vacation, there are new places to explore, sights to see, and things to taste. There will be a larger budget than usual for such things, but I need to be wise and consider the cost, whatever is happening with regard to dollars and points. I need to have some sense about it, because there is a cost. Many times it's worth it for the experience and the memories. When vacation is over, day-to-day life is there. Including the bills. And the scale.

So I think I will be mindful and present when I'm eating and potentially not tracking everything. But whatever the scale says when vacation is done, I'll have my tools for tracking my foods and moods. They will still work. And I know I will still need to use them if I lose weight, stay the same, or gain.

That justification thing stuck in my head for another post.

JUSTIFY FULL-SCALE CONFLICT
June 4, 2012

There are some mixed emotions
For this thing that's called a scale.
It can make a person smile and cheer
Or pout and weep or wail.

It measures what I put on it
Right down to my soles.
It shows me down/up/stay-the-same
No matter what my goals.

And then the justifys can start
As I reflect on what's the truth.

The map unfolds to what I do next
Whether old or in my youth.

I can keep this downtrend going
Just if I keep on using the tools.
I'll stop this uptrend from rising
Just if I slow down and stop the drools.

I would have had a loss I know
Just if I hadn't eaten salt.
I would have gained a whole lot more
Just if I caved and drank a malt.

I know I would have lost even more
Just if I walked or ran miles.
I will continue my journey to health
Just if I keep on through trials.

I'll keep a steady maintenance
Just if I have healthy fear
Of throwing all my hard work away.
Just if I lose my WW gear.

Some folks weigh once weekly.
I weigh at least once a day.
I do what works for my success
And that's perfectly okay.

The scale is not really my enemy
To be faced with fear and dread.
But rather a patient faithful friend
Just if I settle it first in my head!

With all my thinking and planning and writing, there came a time to actually go on vacation. Here's my last post before leaving the East Coast for the West Coast.

POINTING FROM A DIFFERENT DIRECTION
June 23, 2012

I'm headed out on vacation
To a far out western point.
I'm going to use my non-tech tools

And practice what I've loint.

And so upon this beautiful morn
With a low number on the scale
I decided to make it official
For the start of my vacay tale.

I could have had a buffer—
A one-point-six-pound slide—
But as a show of what happened next
I couldn't let it ride.

So in this my swan song poetry
Before I duck this coast
I have a little barnyard rhyme
To encourage me, at the most.

I won't be grazing all day long
And moo-reen like a cow
Or wallowing in mud (of self-pity)
Like her porcine friend the sow.

I'll race around
But not eat like a horse.
I'll try new things
Not be chicken, of course.

My limits on sugar are for my brain
Not for a quick weight-loss crown.
But I'm happy to say
On vacation day
My weight is significantly down!

My victory on the scale before going on vacation didn't send me into the overconfidence mode that tripped me up at Gettysburg. I went on vacation with a plan and a purpose to enjoy my time.

POST-VACATION POST
July 7, 2012

First of all. Just to get back into the swing of things, the capital letters in my title spell *point*. That's the point. Here I am back at my post, posting points on my blog and on my tracker. I weighed myself this morning, and I was the same as when I weighed in two weeks ago. I think that's pretty good.

I stayed the same
And I'm pleased as punch.
I didn't e-track
Breakfast, dinner, or lunch.
I did what I could
And kept true to my plan
No grazing between meals
Nor sweets, such as flan.

That brings me to a story about flying from New York City to Seattle via Minneapolis. As we backed out from the gate at Minneapolis, the power went off. Lights out. Engine off. The public address announcement: "Flight attendants, switch to manual mode." It was a little disconcerting, but I had this funny mental image of all the windows opening, arms reaching out, and us flapping our way to Seattle. That didn't happen. The engines started, and we were on our merry way. I drank lots of water. I picked the snack my daughter enjoyed and gave it to her. *And.*

How about a drumroll here?
A noteworthy victory.
I fit easily into the lav
When I had to … (use it)!

I had forgotten that it would still be daylight when we landed in Seattle—even though it was 9:15 p.m. We had the special treat of flying by Mount Rainier with the sun shining on it. It was like a gift. My grandmother did paintings of that mountain. My husband and I and our three kids hiked there after my grandmother's funeral. My uncle and several cousins have climbed Mount Rainier. Another uncle's house has a beautiful view of it. And there it was. Welcome to Washington and the 2012 family reunion!

I won't go into all the little details, but there's the first story. It's so fitting for my journey with WW tools. On manual mode. Lots of activity. Doing what works.

Our vacation started with a tour of the Olympic Peninsula, but then it was time to meet up with the rest of the family for the reunion.

EAST OF THE CASCADES
July 10, 2012

On our recent vacation, we headed from the Pacific Coast over the Cascades into central Washington. Past farm lands. And then past sage brush and windmills and lots of open spaces with very few trees. The Columbia River Gorge. Dry waterfalls. The Grand Coulee Dam. Mesas. Plateaus. Black-tailed deer. Cherry stands. The town of George. We stopped for ice cream at a little store. I got an Oscar Meyer snack pack and had Rainier cherries along with the cheese and turkey rounds. Metal horse sculptures at Vantage. We finally arrived at Kettle Falls where the rest of the family was waiting for us at three very large houseboats.

We stayed in the marina that night. Made a Wal-Mart run. Had grilled salmon, asparagus, green beans, and brown rice/quinoa mix in abundance. Reconnected with cousins. Went on another Wal-Mart run in the morning. And then we were off! Going north on the dammed-up Columbia River that is called Lake Roosevelt. Beautiful. Happy. Content. Not thinking about food!

I had one little blip. Someone saw me walking with a handful of cherries after supper (I considered it part of my supper—I was just walking to the car for the first Wal-Mart run). She said, "Are you *still* eating?" I don't know if she had noticed I had lost a significant amount of weight since the last reunion. But it used to be that comments like that would knock me for a loop and into a binge. I noticed it. And moved on. I mention it because it was a victory for me.

I'll not go into all the details of the reunion. It was a very special time. I have some amazing relatives. And I felt like I was one of them! I had great conversations. I helped prepare good food when it was my assigned time. And I helped other teams when it was appropriate.

I ate three meals a day. I didn't eat desserts—not even the ones I concocted. I was satisfied with the sights and smells and compliments. And it was good. No cravings. Several explanations. Praise for the WW tools and *Potatoes Not Prozac* when it was appropriate.

I had a great time with great folks. And then it was time to head home. Tired, happy, and thankful. No weight gain or post-vacation binge. Just a lot of great memories. Some involve food. But they don't revolve around food.

It seems fitting that this vacation encompassed Independence Day.

I had proof that I could be me in a vacation experience. I wasn't controlled by food or sugar. I wasn't obsessed with missing my online tools. I was present when I was there. And when I got home, I was present there too.

NUMBERS
July 12, 2012

This weekend, there's a high likelihood that people who haven't seen me for a while will tell me I shouldn't lose any more weight. There's a chance some people will say I'm too thin. I'm in a better place than I've ever been to handle comments like that. My blood work numbers are good. I'm close to my healthy weight. And that's what I'll mind (pay attention to).

The reason I didn't stay at my goal weight before wasn't because it was too low. It was because of my sugar addiction. I know from experience, and the science in *Potatoes Not Prozac*, that I have to be super careful with sugar. Just about like a recovering alcoholic has to be with alcohol. And with that knowledge, I'm going to keep using the tools, including Maintenance. When it's right. When it's time. Lifetime.

Eureka! Some of my ideas surprised me with their simple but profound discoveries.

BRAINSTORM
July 25, 2012

Yesterday, I noticed that *eat* was a part of creativity. And in that moment, I felt like I had discovered something exciting. I had been a bit off with my blogging. And it occurred to me that I do better with creativity in my day.

I am a creative cook. I look at cookbooks, google recipes, and study menus. And I cook. Sometimes I attempt to follow recipes. And sometimes I get interesting results.

One time I was determined to follow a dinner plan I'd signed up for online. The dinner of the day was Tarragon Chicken, but when I started in on the recipe, I found out I didn't have tarragon or chicken in my house. There wasn't time to run to the store, so I followed the recipe with what I had. We ate Marjoram Pork that night.

When we were houseboating on Lake Roosevelt, I made bread pudding with leftover toasted hamburger buns, Good Earth Sweet and Spicy Tea, hot apple cider mix, eggs, and milk. I did something similar with leftover rice and quinoa for pudding. And when the pears started getting overripe, I turned them into apearantly apple crisp with instant oatmeal and butter.

Back to the creative thing. I have discovered that I do better when I have a creative outlet. And instead of playing with food, I think it's probably better all the way around (and I'm not as far around as I used to be) if I play with words! There is a certain creativity with food. Artistry for the palate and the plate. But someone usually has to eat it, and sometimes that's a problem. With words, it's best if you don't eat them.

Even though this wasn't the beginning of my blog, I got into an initial phase.

THE ABCS AND A D
August 1, 2012

Aware: This is huge in my weight-loss journey, soon to be my healthy-weight journey. I am aware of what I eat and how I am feeling. I am aware of sugar being dangerous for me. I am, ah, where I need to be—online for support (when I can) and noticing how my surroundings are affecting me (or not). I am "a weigher" of food and myself. This works for me. And I'm thankful.

Beware: I've noticed that I need to be extra careful when I am tired, stressed (desserts backward), or not able to measure and track my food and weight. Sugar lurks in strange places, and if I think it might be in something, I stay away from it. And if I can't stay away from it for some strange reason, I make sure I have protein to go with it. I do this because I've found that sugar controls me if I'm not controlling it. I need to remember to be where I am. That's being present. It's a nice gift.

C (see) Where: I think it's a good idea to see where I've been, where I am, and where I want to be. The online tools keep a record of what I've eaten, how I've felt, and what I've weighed. I can also see where my friends have been, where they are now, and where they are going. It's good.

De-wear: I am getting rid of the clothes that are too big for me. Or that I just don't like.

And with that, I got to the post where I reached my healthy-weight range! I had been logging, jogging, and blogging for just over seven months. I had been using my WW *tools with my* Potatoes Not Prozac *rules.*

STANDARD POINT

August 8, 2012

This morning I weighed myself and saw that I had reached my healthy-weight range! I haven't been able to track my foods or blog over the last week, but I've kept an active awareness of what's been going on in my mind and also what's going into my mouth.

This week my weight also dropped below that of my husband. I take notice of that not because I'm in competition with him or because I base my weight on his. Not anymore, anyway. I am realizing that for years I figured if I weighed ten or twenty pounds less than him, I was okay. I'm an inch shorter than he is, and that made sense to me. Over the years (not counting three pregnancies), that was how I thought about my weight.

And then I passed him. I'd think, *Oh, it's only ten pounds.* And then twenty and so on. There were some yo-yo fluctuations, but for years, I was heavier than he was. He has been very loving and supportive of me no matter what my weight. And I appreciate that.

My tendency has been to gain weight if anyone has made any comments about my heaviness. Or my thinness. Or whatever. I think that mind-jerk reaction had a lot to do with my sugar addiction.

This time down, though, I am very aware that I'm not on a diet. I'm not comparing myself to other people and their journeys. I'm working this to be healthy. That is the standard, and there is something wonderful about that!

I haven't been blogging or logging much in the past week. That will probably be how it goes for the next couple of weeks.

I've been away from my normal routine, and my keen focus has been more on spiritual things. This blog isn't about that. I'll just say I've appreciated a verse from Isaiah 55 that says, "Wherefore do ye spend money for that which is not bread? and your labour for that which satisfieth not? hearken diligently unto me, and eat ye that which is good, and let your soul delight itself in fatness."

There are a lot of analogies. What I focus (or feed) on in my mind, spirit, or body has a direct impact on the health of each of those aspects of what is me—positives, thankfulness, pure things. It has a lot to do with choices. Fatness is good for my soul but not for my body.

I've seen a lot of people recently who I haven't seen for a year or more. I'm at least fifty pounds lighter than when they last saw me. I've gotten a lot of positive comments. And I've gotten a lot of questions about how I lost so much weight. I've been told I'm a shadow of myself. My standard response is: "This is me. I just don't have the excess anymore. I changed some things about how I eat, and the excess weight has gone away—sort of a side effect."

People started asking me for pointers on how to lose weight.

POINTERS
August 22, 2012

What do I say when someone wants to know how I lost so much weight? I hesitate to tell people I'm on WW. When I mention WW, the response is often: "Oh. WW. I lost a lot of weight on that diet years ago, but then they changed the points values and I hated it." I know exactly what they are talking about. I lost a bunch of weight on that diet quite a few times. And I gained it and more back each time. When they changed the program, I rebelled and gained the weight back.

This time, *I* changed. I changed the way I think about sugar. I changed the way I eat. I use the WW tools for tracking. I make sure I'm eating enough. I make sure I eat healthy foods. I connect with friends who are also using tools that I use. I log my food, jog my move, and blog my moods. And the excess weight goes away.

I kept returning to my initial phase, but it wasn't starting over again. I was continuing to do what was working for me.

H.O.P.E.
August 23, 2012

There's something wonderful about hope. It starts me where I am and helps me in a positive direction.

The word came to me this morning, and I thought about each letter in several ways with regard to using the WW tools.

Helping Obese People Excell. Yes, I know excel is spelled with one *L*. But I'm talking about getting rid of cells. When I started this journey, I was wearing size-twenty-two skirts. I've been using the tracking tools faithfully. Last week I was able to wear one of my daughter's size-fours. I think it's safe to say I've gotten rid of a few cells. I put some knit capris on this morning. When I used to use them for Jazzercise a few years ago, they were skintight. This morning, they were loose and flapping in the breeze as I ran a mile. I'm out of my prison cell.

Helping Overweight People Extinguish. Bad habits, like wildfires, need to be put out. I've lost weight before, but bad habits have helped me find it, and more, sooner or later. I put out my habits of excess sugar and grazing between meals before I joined WW. Blogging about my experience has helped reinforce what works for me. And it is continuing to work for me.

Helping Ordinary People Eat. This covers everyone. The tools are designed for life. I joined WW online because I wanted to make sure I ate enough to lose weight. I'm continuing WW online because I want to stay in my healthy-weight range by tracking my foods and moods.

Hope and guilt don't seem to have much of a connection. Weight-loss plans are fueled by hope only to be bogged down by guilt when things don't go as planned. I would read other bloggers' accounts of slipups and shame. And sometimes I struggled with my own slips. I found it helpful to find positives to focus on. This time was in rhyme.

SO WHAT ABOUT GUILT?
September 10, 2012

One thing I like about my plan
Is that it isn't built
On feeling bad about oneself
And wallowing in guilt.

No matter what the starting weight
And how the scale might tilt
Or if, to be in healthy range for height
Means climbing on a stilt.

This collection of tools isn't just about weight
Although they have helped me be thinner.
The support and encouragement within and without

Have convinced me I'm really a winner.

So what about guilt?
It makes me wilt.
Clogs my thinking a little like silt.
It cracks foundations on which I have built.

As far as guilt from eating goes,
Take it away
Learn from the past
But today's a new day.

Sure the scale may go up
If I've just had too much
Or the time of the month
Or so on and such.

But the guilt that can lead to a wallowing binge
That stresses the fridge door off at the hinge
And then makes me, with points, feel stingier than stinge
Needs to be burned up—not just singed.

I learned late last year
I had sugar to fear—
It messes with my brain.
And, while shedding a tear,
I then took courage and cheer—
My weight-loss failures explained.

Since coming to grips
With what padded my hips
I've been careful with what goes in.
Sure, I've slipped a few times
(In documented rhymes)
And I've taken it on the chin.

But guilt isn't what has saved me
And gotten me back on track.
It's thankfulness. Knowing what I can do
To counter sugar's attack.

The memory of how it used to be
When I simply had no control
The headaches I had when I detoxed

Get me back on a roll.

It's three meals a day with some protein
Not grazing right through like a cow.
Actively living with tracking tools
Not wallowing in guilt like a sow.

I'm at peace with my program
And how it's working for me.
I'm headed right into lifetime
And happily feeling free!

Several days later, I was having trouble with food. I wanted to be cured of sugar addiction or sensitivity so I wouldn't have to be so careful of it all the time. But my reality is that I am sensitive to sugar, and if I am not careful, I have to deal with it before it takes control over me.

TALKING MYSELF THROUGH
September 18, 2012

I'm feeling a little lousy.
It's raining cats and dogs.
Yes, I'm feeling rather out of sorts.
I think I should read some blogs.

I had my lunch at eleven.
And then a two-hour nap.
When I awoke I had more to eat.
My dailies were gone in a snap.

Yes, it's one of those ornery days
The kind that sometimes come
And make me feel like eating everything
For a food-hazed mind-dulled numb.

'Twould have been better to focus on blogs, I think
Before I filled up on food.
Read about struggles and weight-loss success
Instead of my I-don't-care mood.

But what's done is done and this too shall pass.
I know that for a fact.
The sky's getting brighter, my mood will grow lighter

And the food I ate has been tracked.

The lesson I think I can take away
From this ordinary but ornery day
Is if the sky is overcast grey
I should turn the lights on inside.

Excess food doesn't make me light.
(Au contraire, it makes me a fright.)
And before I take another big bite,
Check, "Am I trying to hide?"

Facing up to what's going on
Is half of the battle won
So I'll continue this journey that I've begun
A winner, because I have tried.

Part of my former weight-loss struggle was not sticking with programs and not keeping the weight off. Nothing I did seemed sustainable. After nine months of working my tools, I could feel like I was sustaining my efforts to be healthy. Hence, this next post.

SUSTAINED APPLAUSE
September 25, 2012

I've been working my weight-management tools from the try-angle, and I've had great results. I'm going for sustained, because everything I'm doing is with lifetime in mind. I've lost weight before. I've been on diets and more diets. I've been applauded, but it hasn't been sustained. I'm not really looking for sustained applause. I'm looking for sustained results.

I've been under stress. I've been on vacation. I've been sick. I've been healthy. I've been happy. I've been sad. I've been silly. And I've been serious. I have mourned. I have rejoiced. And I've sustained my use of the tools. I have kept to my eating plan. I have written blog posts. I have read and commented on regular and random blogs. I have interacted with "old" friends online. I've made new friends online. I've taken full-scale snapshots of my weight. I've recognized non-scale victories. I've walked. I've run. I've raced. It's fun.

I've resisted trying exercise programs that I didn't think I would sustain. I've opted for walking with a friend in the mornings. I've found that I enjoy running, so I'm doing that too. If I get to the point of joining a gym, it will be because I want to not because I think I should. I want what I do to be sustainable.

When I started blogging, I worried a little that I couldn't keep coming up with things to write about. But because I'm writing about my life, there is always something. Maybe it's not always exciting. But there is always something, because I keep at it. And it keeps working.

I get into rhyming mode every once in a while. And if my thoughts come out that way, that's what I say. I don't refrain from it. But I don't feel like I have to sustain that mode of writing. And if I have a play on words that amuses me, I go for it. Sometimes the puns are unintended. Sometimes I get fan mail for my brain!

And as an addendum (*dum* de *dum* drumroll): I sustained a run for five miles this afternoon. But there was no applause. Because my thighs don't clap anymore!

Life has its regularities. And sometimes they're not so regular. Lack of fiber, lack of sleep, lack of exercise, or various other factors can affect regularity. It's not something I talk about very much, but it's a fact of life that I had to deal with at times.

BALANCE POINT
September 27, 2012

Yesterday I was full of prunes.
This morning, I am not.
I haven't had to run real fast
But more of a focused trot.

I think the lesson here for me
Is balance in life and on scale.
Paying attention to fiber and diet
And living to tell the tale.

The use of the D-word is qualified
I'm not on a diet, per se—
It's paying attention and using my tools—
Living it every day.

As a sugar addict, there's a balance to being aware of the dangers that lurk in foods and being able to just live life. It's so much easier when it's not all about food.

KEEPING FIT
September 27, 2012

I parked at the library when I went for a three-mile run this morning. When I finished my run, I headed into the library. A man got to the door just as I was approaching, and he kindly and politely held it open for me. I thanked him, and he said, "Didn't I just see you running along the street?"

I said, "Yes!"

And he said, "It's great to keep fit!"

To *keep* fit! I'm thinking that means he thought I looked like I *was* fit!

I'm having a flashback to returning some exercise DVDs a couple of years ago. The fellow at the check-in counter said, "And how did these work for you?"

Uh. I had to tell him the truth. I never opened the case.

Another time, I remember actually sitting in a chair to watch a walking DVD I had bought. But *now*, I'm a runner!

And then there were the days when the old habits were closer to the surface than I realized.

EXECUTE EXCUSE
September 28, 2012

I nearly ate a handful of peanuts earlier this afternoon. Not because I was hungry. Not because I needed them. Not even because I wanted them. It was just because they were there. I had them in my hand. I was poised to crack open the first shell, but I put them back in the container. There was no excuse and no reason to eat them, so I didn't.

Now instead of having to log in points of no return (although they would surely return on my hips), I am blogging about not having to. And I'm feeling pleased that I chose not to.

I think one of the things that saved me was a pair of tights I'm wearing today. Yesterday, I saw some tights I liked and decided to buy them. But first, I needed to get the right size. Last year I was cramming my legs into the largest size and having to buy tights fairly often because they were too tight and tended to spring runs even though it was fall. This year I'm reading the label on the next smaller size and finding out I really need one smaller than that.

I realize that in order to sustain this smaller size, I need to pay attention. I know I still have the capability to eat like a fat person. I'm thin right now, and if I want to stay that way, I'll eat like a thin person on purpose. Three meals a day, and no grazing.

And even if the excuse is a cute one, it doesn't fit in my eating style. Ex a cute excuse.

Although I usually had a lot to say when I wrote, sometimes just a few words worked just fine.

THE TALL, SKINNY ONE
September 30, 2012

A friend of mine told me this morning that if someone were describing me, that's what they could say.

Pun alert. Enough said.

THE BEST OF THE WURST
October 1, 2012

Here it is: a brand-new month.
The date: October first.
It can be the best month yet
Or it could be the wurst.

I'm not inclined to Oktoberfest
But I once sau sage advice.
For every thing I want to eat
I prob'bly should think twice.

The beer part's not a temptation.
I simply have never imbibed.
It plain old doesn't interest me

No matter how it's described.

It is the season to bulk up
If I had to hibernate.
But I'm actually planning to stay alert
To maintain my lifetime weight.

So I'll likely just smell frankfurters
Boiled, grilled, or fried.
And that will take care of the wurst of it
Don't knack it till you've tried.

If I were feeling a bit deprived
And wanted to indulge.
I'd make sure I counted every bite
To prevent a waistline bulge.

My attitude's not meant to be
Spoiled or even brat-ty.
I just think this sausage stuff
Is entirely way too fatty.

I'm not sure what all was happening at the time, but this invitation was to a pity party. There can be a dangerous let-down period after a bout of success. It's hard to explain, but it's very real. Writing helped me send regrets to this pity party instead of experiencing them.

INVITE TO A PARTY
October 2, 2012

An invite to a party
But it doesn't sound like fun
For this particular party
Has room enough for one.

This party isn't dress up.
It's "come just as you are."
It's not to lift my spirits
But to drag them down real far.

No. This party is a pity.
A real down in the dump.
It's best to find an excuse to not go

Or get a kick in the rump.

The food isn't really special
But it always can be found.
Its siren song is to make me feel good
But it only makes me round.

I'm writing up this little rhyme
Then getting out of my chair
Staying away from that party for one.
I can't afford to be there.

There is oh so much to be thankful for
And it's best I focus on that.
Instead of pity-partying on
I'm out of here and stat!

There's a fine line between encouragement and discouragement. My reaction in this situation was probably a warning sign of addictive behavior. Awareness was my key to turning it around.

A COUPLE OF POINTS
October 3, 2012

I considered going for a run this morning before my official weigh-in. My husband asked me if I really wanted to because it would make it hard for next week. I just looked at him and said, "I have been working this for almost a year. I think I know what I'm doing." And that was fine. But I decided to just record the number I saw first thing this morning. Because, in my mind, that really finished off last week. I needed it to be over.

This is a brand-new week. I have all my points reset. I have my eating plan. I have my exercise plan. And I'm blogging.

Last week was tough. But it's over. This week is now. And I'm on it.

As I read through these entries, I remember the struggle with sugar. It's a reality that I live with. I also remember feeling like a failure. I had been encouraged to write a book of my experiences, but when I had slipups with sugar, I felt like a fraud. Who would want to read about failure? But then I realized it wasn't failure if I kept trying. And that's what this is about. Later I would understand better that sugar sensitivity isn't something that can be fixed. It's something to live with. That's what I do.

TRUE CONFESSIONS
October 5, 2012

I'm not sure what happened
But I really came unhinged.
I cracked and succumbed.
You could say that I have binged.

That's not the search engine
Of non-Google fame
But uncontrolled eating
That makes my good health lame.

I'll not hide this folly.
It's a matter of fact.
I put food in my mouth.
It was my own act.

I knew that it wasn't
Part of my plan
But I ate it in spite or
To spite—should have ran.

So now I am feeling
Not very okay
Because I really OD'd
On sugar today.

It's been quite a while
But I know the score.
It's time to be real
Not time to have more.

I'm back on track.
Not a moment to spare.
Can't wait for tomorrow
To get back to care.

For whatever the reason
I can't quite explain
I let too much sugar
Into my brain.

Perhaps I was testing
Is this really true?
Can't I have just a taste
With no hullabaloo?

Well, yet once again
I've proved what is wrong
And I'll have to keep singing
My no-sugar song.

It doesn't have to be
Sung like the blues.
It's not sad and mopey
It's just what I do-s.

My plan simply works
When I just use my tools
Today I didn't.
I feel like three fools.

Enough of the rhyming.
I'm going to bed.
And I'll pull all the covers
Right over my head.

Tomorrow is coming.
I'm planning to run.
I'll work all my tools
Until I am done.

The recovery didn't always go smoothly, but I didn't quit. At some point I would crave feeling better more than the next sugar hit and crash.

WHY DO I DO THIS?
October 8, 2012

We had a potluck lunch at our house yesterday. There was a wonderful group of people and a nice assortment of food. I fixed sausage (hot and sweet) and peppers (and tomatoes and onions). I cooked the sausages in the Crock-Pot on Saturday and drained the fat before I added the peppers, onions, and tomatoes. I made breadsticks with spinach, garlic, Italian seasonings, and parmesan cheese. I also served corn off the cob—yummy without salt or butter. I had roasted, cut, and frozen it last summer.

On Saturday afternoon, my husband had picked up some local apples at a farm stand. When I went to put them in the fridge, I noticed a few that needed to be used right away. So I made an apple dessert. It would have been fine to slice and bake them with a little cinnamon. But no. I sliced them; sprinkled them with cinnamon; topped them with a mixture of butter, sugar, flour, and egg; and baked them. Bad idea.

I did fine with lunch. One plateful. Small helpings of a potato/ham casserole, stuffed shells, buttercup squash, salad, sausage, another casserole with rice, and half of a breadstick. I ate a fresh macoun apple for dessert. I admired the triple-layer chocolate cake, the pumpkin pie, the ice cream, the caramel corn, and my own apple dessert. But I didn't have any. And our guests took the leftovers home. (*You take the cake!*)

Suppertime came along. I was hungry. I wanted pizza, and I decided to make some. Because it takes time to make the dough and get the oven to temp, I decided to see if there were some justifiable way to try the apple dessert I made. There wasn't any sugar in the sliced apples themselves. It was just on the topping. And so I dug in. And then I didn't care quite so much if there was a little topping mixed in. It wasn't pretty. It tasted okay, but I think it could be likened to doing drugs or alcohol for me. Because I started looking for more hits. And they were there.

This morning was fine. And then I had the idea to use up some leftover coffee (Peet's Major Dickinson Blend) from the potluck. And some leftover half-and-half (I had about a quart that needed to be used or tossed). I should have dumped it all. But I didn't. I made caramels. Mocha caramels. With the intent of not even tasting them.

When the caramels were done, I poured them into a buttered pan, spilling just a couple of drops on the counter. Like a crack addict, I swooped the spillage up with one finger and tasted it. Bad idea. I'll not go into the rest of the details. It would have been better to throw out the coffee and half-and-half.

Even though I waxed poetic about getting right back on my plan after having a problem last week, I'm back there again after having done extremely well since last November. But I need to notice that there are only a few documented cases of me slipping up and getting back on track. The most famous was the Battle of Gettysburger. It lasted three days.

I'm not sure if this will be a named battle. I could call it the Fall of Maurlean? *No.* I may have tripped up, but it's just autumn. I'm not going with the fall. I am convinced I have to treat sugar seriously. Similar to how a recovering alcoholic has to treat alcohol. And I'm on the one-minute-at-a-time-I'll-get-through-this step.

I finally reached the point of horror. I was barely holding on to my tools to deal with sugar. I certainly wasn't using them effectively. Here's what happened next.

WAKING UP
October 9, 2012

This morning I weighed myself. And I got an eye-opener way more effective than coffee. I discovered I was ten pounds heavier than what I weighed last Tuesday. Theoretically (and I am *not* out to prove it), I could gain eighty pounds back in eight weeks.

Ate weaks. That's how I would do it. Sugar weakens my impulse controls. And over the last week, culminating (cul*max*eating) with yesterday's fatsidiots food frenzy comple*at* with all kinds of things that I will not list here in case it could cause problems for anyone reading this (or writing this), I have found some pounds that I thought I wasn't looking for. But I ate like I was searching for them like gold. Unlike gold, though, they were pretty easy to find.

Although I am very aware that I am human, I am now aware that my online friends are aware I am human. And it's okay. It's more than okay. It's the tools at work. Working. Thank you very much. For your care and kindness. For your comments.

So I'm awake. And I have a plan that I've already started to execute, because I don't want to kill my successful weight loss and being healthy.

This morning: I dropped my daughter off at school, and then I went for a three-mile run from the grocery store to where the sidewalk ends and back. As an aside, there's a horseshoe nailed to the telephone pole where the sidewalk ends. Some people might think of it as good luck, but I think of it as a turnaround sign. Today, it stood for a double turnaround. Not in the sense of full circle. I'm not wanting to resemble that again. I'm just thinking turnaround for my feet and turnaround for my defeat.

When I got back to the store, I went in to look for some gluten-free pie crust mix that I need to make a gluten-free pie for a friend's son's wedding (I won't be there, so I won't be eating it). I made my loop by the seafood department and spotted a manager's special lobster roll for three dollars. I decided to get it. But I also decided to not eat it until I got home and transferred the lobster to a whole-grain tortilla and added salad greens to it. That's a non-scale victory for me, thank you very much.

I made a quick stop at home to shower and change, make the sandswitch (new word), and headed out to do a few errands.

My first stop was the WW center. I've been in healthy range for a few weeks, but I've put off the lifetime reactivation process, because I'm not sure why. This morning I decided I was not going to wait for my weight to be any lower or higher. I had the option to raise my goal weight because of my age. And that was in this morning's plan. No games. Just do it.

I was delayed because of road paving, but I was not to be deterred. And then it took me three phone calls to WW for the receptionist to be able to weigh me in and process my material. I wanted a guarantee that my blog/online materials would not be altered in any way. (I had read some horror stories about that happening.) My cell phone beeped low battery, and I had a Bluetooth problem when I went out to my car to plug the phone in so I wouldn't drop the call. None of it weakened my resolve. And I succeeded in carrying out my plan. I weighed in under goal. And I plan to be lower next week when I get my voucher for free eTools. I'm feeling lighter already.

Yes. The tools work when I use them. The scale is one of those tools. And although it doesn't work for everyone to use that tool every day, it works for me. I have to treat this healthy living thing as a full-scale war. There may be casualties from time to time. I'm pretty sure this time they were caused by casual lies. About sugar. About mealtimes versus grazing. About weighing.

Awareness and action are part of the healing process. And once again, I'm back. Enthusiastically.

Although I already knew writing about my feelings was a big part of my way to deal with my sugar addiction, I was more convinced than ever that it worked for me.

ADDICTION POINT
October 10, 2012

I'm not certain at just which point
Addiction's the diagnosis

But this I know
Sure as the nose I blow
Recovery is in my prognosis.

Recovery can be a definite thing
That can firmly be put in one's past
Or it can be
(As it is for me)
A day-by-day process to last.

I've documented in prose and in rhyme
My journey of weight loss and health.
I've sounded the trumpet
That sugar's the culprit
In crystalline form or in stealth.

WW has helped me be healthy
With wonderful tool after tool.
It's not a diet.
It's living—just try it!
It works, and there's no one to fool.

Back to addiction: I had no prediction
That comments to blogs I would crave.
I write up a post
More often than most
And I love a response to my rave!

That's part of what WW is about
Community and people that care.
Jean Nidetch was right:
When your clothes are too tight
It's easier to lose when you share!

So I'll continue to write and do what's right.
Use the tools how they work for me.
Read and comment on blogs.
Track my food, mood, and jogs
Through my lifetime goal of healthy!

I had learned to value exercise when I took up jogging, and I wanted to make sure I had something to do if the weather put up a roadblock.

EXERCISE POINTS

October 11, 2012

I used to go to Jazzercise classes quite a bit, but I ended up quitting a couple of summers ago when I just got tired of the music. It was getting into my head and popping up when I didn't want it to. It seemed time to give it a rest. I got a notice in the mail yesterday, and I decided to rejoin today. I've been getting a good amount of exercise running and walking, but I've noticed a need to do some upper-body stuff.

I was a bit late this morning, but I got the lights green and the class started late. I missed a little of the warm-up, but I got my own version of a warm-up by putting on my socks and shoes while I was filling out the registration forms and paying. I got out into the gym to find that my feet remembered the moves, and it felt good. I felt good.

Because I have taken another healthy step for myself, I have a plan for when the sidewalks are frozen over. I have a plan for my core and upper arms. I'm not planning how to treat myself after class. The class is the treat. And that is the point!

REACHING A HEALTHY WEIGHT

Still Working on My Mind

Although the number on the scale indicated healthy, I knew I still had work to do to in my head. I couldn't let a number on the scale keep me from my ultimate goal of overall healthy.

FREE
October 16, 2012

I am writing today as a free lifetime member of WW. I got my lifetime status more than twenty years ago. But I didn't take care of it, and I lost it because I gained weight. And then I didn't weigh in because of the gain. I gained because I stopped using the tools. I gained because I hadn't broken free of my poor eating habits. I gained because I was addicted to sugar and didn't know it. (I actually suspected it, but I didn't know what to do about it.) I gained because my goal had been a number and not a lifetime of healthy. I gained because even though I said differently, I used WW as a diet. I didn't see a plan for the rest of my life. And so I found and gained back all the weight I had lost plus a lot more.

I've lost a lot of weight this year. I'm more than eighty pounds lighter than I was at my highest measured weight. But not too long ago, I found I was very capable of gaining it all back. Boom. Ten pounds in one week. I was still in my healthy range, but I had a warning and I heeded it.

This past week, I paid close attention to what I was doing. I made sure I followed my plan of reduced sugar and no grazing. I rejoined Jazzercise. I ran a 5K in Hartford. And today when I went to the meeting and weighed in, I was down almost four pounds and *free*.

Yes. I've lost a lot of weight. But I've gained a lot of other things. Control over food. Access to nicer and easier-to-find clothes. Good health. The ability to run six miles for enjoyment. I've gained some self-respect. I've gained a bunch of wonderful and supportive online friends in the WW blogging community. I've gained an appreciation for every single pound (or part of a pound) in both directions on the scale. And more. Not necessarily in that order.

Outside support is a huge help in achieving goals. I was fortunate to have good cheerleaders. My dad was the best.

PA PA POINT
October 17, 2012

This is not about stuttering. Although I have stuttered with weight loss many times. No. This is about my dad. I was going to say father, but I happened to notice that in English, this is also *fat her.* That's what I have been writing about for months in my journey to be thin her.

So. My dad. There isn't enough room to write about him here. But I will say he's an amazing man. He's a smart, funny, artistic (drawing, piano-playing, singing, whistling, meat-carving, and arranging), athletic (hockey, baseball, ping-pong), hard-working (retired small-business owner, lawn cutting, tree cutting, log splitting, house maintaining), sensitive, spiritual, caring, loving man. He's inventive and can fix just about anything with just about nothing. He's a believer in using good tools. And he's a lifetime member of WW.

He loves to read. And he reads my blog. He especially likes to read the comments that people leave for me. He's been in pretty good health, although recently he's had some bumps in the road. His doctors are amazed with his numbers. He's aging, as we all are. He is aware of this life not being a permanent fixture. And he's been preparing for the future.

While I appreciate him for a lot of things, this last thing is the most valuable. And although it's not something I write about a lot in my blog, it is most important to me. And so, I'll just say that I'm glad for all the things in everyday life (including this weight-loss journey) that point to something more. Things that make me pause and consider something bigger and better. A plan. A purpose. And provision.

Nature points to this. Families point to this. They are things that our human minds can grasp and think about to give us a little glimpse or comparison to what is available and what will be on a higher level. Love. Hope. Compassion. Mercy. Forgiveness. Peace. Safety. Comfort. My dad points to this in the way he lives. My mom does too. And I'm thankful.

Not every situation cheers, though. Some are just challenging.

CONTROLLED SUBSTANCE
October 18, 2012

Today I was invited to a friend's home to have coffee, play some games, and have lunch. I was able to decline the cinnamon rolls, cookies, grapes, cheese, and crackers when we had coffee. She had made the rolls and cookies herself. But she knows I don't eat between meals. And she was okay with it.

Lunch was California Tacos. She fries her soft taco shells and serves them filled with seasoned meat and cheese. She had homemade salsa, shredded lettuce, and hot sauce to go with them. I had two tacos—one corn and one wheat. And that was fine.

I had a piece of homemade gluten-free lemon meringue pie for dessert. It was all very sweet. The figurative part was fine, but the literal part was too much for me. And I felt lousy after I ate it. It was one of those situations where I felt like it was better for me to just accept the serving and politely eat it instead of declining it.

I had run two miles this morning after dropping my daughter off at school. I have lost almost all of the ten pounds I gained a couple of weeks ago. I had the points. But the sugar is like a drug to me. I know that WW doesn't limit food choices, but there are things I really shouldn't have.

I am on high alert this afternoon. Well, actually, I felt pretty low for a while. I managed to drive home and track my food before falling asleep on the couch. I seriously could not stay awake any longer. I know it was the sugar. I used to pass out like this when I was out of control with it. I hated that feeling, but I was out of control and I wasn't sure how to regain control. It's days like today that make me so glad for the *Potatoes Not Prozac* book that clued me in to kicking the sugar habit.

I have a headache, but I'm not going to take the easy way out with more sugar. I've proved it's not the easy way at all. It's not the season for snow, but a snowball effect could happen pretty fast. And so I'm blogging instead of eating. I'm talking to myself. I'm remembering what I used to do. And I'm remembering what it did to me. And I'm not going back.

I took a sub stance on the sugar issue today. But it is controlled. Minute by minute. I'm getting through it. With some help from my tools. They work.

I kept writing about my tools working, but recovery wasn't always an instant thing. There were times I wrote blog posts and got lots of encouraging comments from the blogging community. Sometimes that helped right away. And sometimes it took longer. But it always took.

SOMETiMES
October 25, 2012

Sometimes I feel strong and then get whacked with a challenge. And maybe the challenge is better seen as an opportunity to stay strong and use the tools. It doesn't always happen that way. But the idea is nice!

Today I treated myself to a visit with my folks. They live about two hours northeast of me. I've been wanting to visit them for a couple of weeks, but it just didn't work. Today worked.

I stopped at a farm stand on the way and got some winter squash and apples. The produce was beautiful, and the prices were super. There was one variety of squash for ten cents a pound. They looked like giant D'Anjou pears. My mom and I cooked one to see if it was worth getting more on the way home. It wasn't. The seeds I roasted with garlic, salt, rosemary, and coconut oil turned out nice. But it wasn't worth it to get more squash for just the seeds.

My mother fixed paninis on whole-wheat sandwich thins—cheddar cheese, turkey breast, and sweet onion. Served with optional hot pepper jam. And fresh apples and grapes. It was just right. We also sampled the squash but decided to feed it to the compost pile. Had I been in a sugar fog, I might have tried to make a pie or caramels out of it.

We had great conversation, including some discussion of comments on my blog!

I left a little after lunch. I knew my daughter was staying after school, and I needed to pick her up. I stopped at a grocery store to pick up some seltzer flavors we don't seem to have in Connecticut: Boston cream pie, chocolate mint, vanilla pear, and eggnog. And then I had to stop again about an hour from home. I was just too tired. I was listening to Agatha Christie's *Murder on the Orient Express* and realized I wasn't getting all of it. Scary. I got off the highway, took a break, and got a McDonald's Snack Wrap and coffee.

Then I stopped for another break and got a McDonald's cone. Whack. You'd think with all the blogging I've done about sugar, I wouldn't even think of doing such a thing. But I did. I thought it would help me get to where I needed to go.

I got to the high school fine. And I got home fine. By the time I tracked everything I'd eaten today, I realized I'd gone way beyond where I wanted to go! But it's tracked. And I have the opportunity to keep tracking. And to be thankful that even though I didn't feel like I met the challenge in the best way, I got through it.

The reality is that tomorrow is a new day with new points. I have a Jazzercise class to go to in the morning and maybe an opportunity to get in a run to where the sidewalk ends and back. Next week looks like a lot of rain and not much opportunity to run. But there should be opportunities to Jazzercise. And there will be opportunities to track!

October started out with the wurst poem, and perhaps it was fitting for me to end with a scary one. This looks like prose, but it's really a deformed poem.

A POEM FOR THE PROSE
October 31, 2012

I'm a little hesitant to write today. But I think I will do it anyway. Right now I feel good. Just how I should. I had some breakfast and went for a run. Just before Jazzercise. And just for fun.

I ran and I ran past a house that was spooky. With coffins and bones and things that were kooky. A bleach-ed white dog with a raspy-ish bark. 'Twill be more frightening—when it gets dark. I won't be trick-or-treating tonight. And I won't eat candy—no, not one bite. 'Cause I am just off of a sugary high, and to me it's more fitting to call it can-die.

Marshmallow-dramatic? You could call it that. But I'll be sticking to what I have learned. Sugar-hazed fog sets me smack in a bog. I've worked hard for the weight loss I've earned. You know I can't handle and won't hold a candle to healthy without a good plan. WW tools with sugar-sensitive rules. That's how I do it. I can!

This post started out in my head as prose. I started typing, and that's how it goes. Just an occasion, and I arose. Why I do it? I don't really knows. But here it is, plain as the day. Flying along with a poem short or long. Some take off a popular song. WW blogging— just write, no wrong. For folks who are skinny or as big as King Kong. That's what I have to say.

Blogging is good therapy for me. I can write out how I'm feeling and then see it in print. I check back for comments, and the feedback is full of points that I can take note of but don't have to log. Just typing something can help me get my mind around it. And sometimes my mind takes me for a ride, and it's fun.

I've been a little concerned lately about my slips and slides with sugar and on the scale. In the past, I've had trouble with weight-loss reversal. When I've been successful and others around me haven't been, I've found myself gaining a bit to not make them feel so bad. Or when someone is doing well—I've not so much been happy for them, but gained a bit of weight—making them look even better.

A few years ago, I was around someone suffering with anorexia. I found myself packing in the food as if I could help her gain a little weight. I don't know much about it, but I think there's a tendency toward co-dependency in some of this. Rereading what I've written, it seems a little twisted. But I have a feeling there will be people who understand exactly what I'm trying to say.

Perhaps a pun alert is all that is needed for this post too.

FOREIGN POINTS
November 28, 2012

I ventured just a little too far
Wading in De Nial.
I had a clue of my perilous state
When I saw my fat ego smile.

A comment on a recent blog post
Gave me cause to reflect on myself.
Thank you, thank you! My friend!
A real, live WW elf!

What she wrote to me
Was what I've known before.
Sugar is poison—a fact for me.

It only, and always, wants more.

I should have double-checked my brakes
Before going to the store.
To survive I'll keep repeating this
Even if I bore.

So back to the land of De Nial
(Atop the food pyramid)
Trying angles of fats, oils, and sweets.
Who was I trying to kid?

What happens to me with sugar
Is a riddle that's not for a Sphinx.
I know that it gets deep inside of my brain
And affects the way that I thinks.

I look for the sweet stuff, including white bread
And I find that I really don't Cair-o
If it's something to eat: salty, sour, and sweet
I'm not inclined to share. Oh!

Forget serving size: 'E gypped me!
Eating like I want to be large.
If I stayed in the land of De Nial
I'd soon be the size of a barge!

I'm flooding my blog post with all of these thoughts.
I won't say, "Mummy's the word."
I'm no longer shrouding in secrecy
What I thought was (but wasn't) absurd.

Sugar is really like poison to me
Like booze to an alcoholic.
It simply wreaks havoc with impulse controls
And my life turns a little bucolic!

Herds in a pasture grazing all day—
Peaceful, contented sheep.
That's okay for ewe if you like
But the prospects, for me, make me weep.

This fact is what got me started
On my successful journey to health

And I'm needing to guard it ferociously
Because sugar's a master at stealth.

Yes, I'm feeling mighty thankful again
For my friend's well-worded save.
I'm glad to be back at home right here
In lifetime! Free and brave!

Yes, I'm using the tools how they work for me
Thankfully knowing what's what.
No need to be floating a barge in De Nial
In a sugarfied stupor—Tut-Tut!

This phase of my sugar-addiction management continued to serve as a shrink for my mind. Therapy of the rhyming kind.

OWNING UP
November 29, 2012

I think I've tried to take ownership
Of things I can't control.
For no-win situations
But I seemed to make it my goal.

This concept's a little bit fuzzy
I might not know how to explain
But I've had a persistent feeling
Tucked inside my brain.

I can't control the wind or sea
Or even the tides of life
But I can control what goes in my mouth
On fork or spoon or knife.

There are situations around me
I can't change for bad or for good
But that doesn't need to prevent me
From doing just what I should.

Perhaps I could look at it this way:
I've allowed things to try to own me.
Giving these things control of my life—
Not really what it should be.

Behaviors of other people
Types of all kinds of foods
What the weather is doing
Needn't control my moods.

It's not that I can't have compassion
For needs of others—I care.
I don't want it affecting my spirit—
With burdens I simply can't bear.

I can't take ownership of others' success
Or, conversely, their failures to thrive.
What I can do is to stand firm and true
And keep my love alive.

The key is a solid foundation
Something not crumbling with shakes.
Keeping attached to this rock-solid base
Doing whatever it takes.

There are deep implications that go with these thoughts
For my blog, though, I'll stick with weight tracking.
Foundations built deep with my personal tools
Are much more resistant to cracking.

As my base is secure
And its maintenance kept
I can own what is mine
And that, only, accept.

This poem is, well, deep
But not meant to offend.
If I am healthy inside
I'm a better friend.

I'm using the tools
They work and I can
Wish the best for you
As you work out *your* plan.

I'd like to inspire and help other folks
I can't do it by giving a push.
I do what I do that has helped me inside

And shown up with a trim smaller … body.

It's not always easy to change, but when the change is right, it's worth the effort!

CHANGING FOR THE BETTER
December 4, 2012

There's something good about changing things up.
And giving new things a whirl.
I traded my fork for a five-pound weight
To do a bicep curl.

For my twenty cents' worth
It helps paradigm shift
Shakes up the doldrums
And gives me a lift.

Cut out the things
That impede my success.
Clean up my cupboards.
Don't live in a mess!

I change my blog up
From poems to prose.
Whatever my brain does
That's how it goes.

Switching to Shakespearian
From rhymes meant for youth
Just because
Or maybe for Seuth.

I considered lots of things in my head. Sometimes the timing was rhyming, and sometimes it was reason.

A POINT ABOUT TIMING
December 5, 2012

This thing that I do with my word
The rhyming that borders absurd.
Has helped me lose weight
Just in time, not too late

And works better than fat-free cheese curd.

I think of a thing that I want to say
And up pops a word of rhyme right away.
The phrasing and timing that comes to my head
Is sometimes quite welcome and not met with dread.

My rhyming seems quite dependent on phrasing and pauses, and if I can interrupt the wave of timing, I can break out of it. I'm not sure what the initial cause is. But it's helping me be creative and giving me things to put in my blog. The creative part is a huge thing for me.

Back to this point about timing. I sometimes wish my timing on getting my eating under control had happened earlier. But then I realize that wish is ridiculous, because there is absolutely no way that can be changed. A better thing for me to focus on is what I can do in the time I have. Which is now. And things that I do now can help my future. Whatever that is. And however long it might be.

That helps me realize the timing is right to notice good things about right now. I've been in weight-loss mode for a year. My official goal weight has been met. I'm actually under it by a few pounds. I'm not sure what my heart goal weight is, but I don't need to be beating myself up about eating. Sure I registered a five-pound gain on the scale yesterday. But it doesn't mean I'm bad. I made some weight-boosting choices in my eating last week, and they showed up on the scale.

The scale doesn't register that I made a lot of changes in my thinking. And it doesn't know that I could fit into a skirt that I hadn't been able to wear even when I was a lower weight. It doesn't calculate that I have less body fat, and that means I'm occupying a smaller amount of space. (Contrary to popular belief, muscle doesn't weigh more than fat, it just takes up less space.)

So back to the beginning of my post. Phrasing and pauses. Or maybe phasing and pauses. I never thought of weight loss or maintenance as being poetic. But perhaps there is a bit of rhythm to it. More freestyle than with form, but it has shaped up nicely as I've stuck with it. My style of poetry is sometimes all over the place. I used to be a little concerned that it didn't make sense. But the bigger thought here is that it works for me. And that's what this is about.

Sometimes one good thought leads to another. The bites, licks, and tastes in my definition of microeconomics was worth looking at again.

JUST A LiTTLE THiNG
December 12, 2012

I'm glad I ever realized
That Bites, Licks, and Tastes do matter
'Cause it was grazing that was messing me up
And heading me toward fatter.

It's best to track those BLTs
Eaten in secret or plain sight
Facing up and being aware
Morning, noon, and night!

Sure those little things alone
Are worth not much more than nil
But consider that the largest whale
Maintains by eating krill.

It all adds up
And it's good for the whale
But that much for me
Is a very sad tale.

I've learned to stop grazing
And eating with sugar.
I've lost many pounds
And gained vim and vigor!

Just as a reminder to me, and to anyone who might stop in and read this first, I liked to revisit why and how I was doing what I was doing with a blog.

REFLECTiON
December 13, 2012

In just a little reflection (my reflection is smaller these days), I'm thinking it's good to take a look into history to see where I used to be and what has helped me get to where I am (healthy-weight range) and where I'm going (for lifetime).

In my past attempts with WW, I found myself resenting trackers, meetings, and fellow meeting goers. I generally had a bad attitude. Sure, I'd lose some weight, but it didn't stay off. And the resulting gain would usually be a new high.

This time, I've embraced the online community and used the tools to work for me. I read blogs and comment on them. Some I follow on a regular basis, and some I randomly pick from what comes up on the list of blogs. I can have my own WW meeting whenever I need it. I write blog posts as I need to.

Some are short. Some are long.
Some are essays. Some mimic song.

I blog when I'm hungry.
Or when I am sad.
I blog when I'm excited.
And feeling rather glad.

It is a creative outlet
And a venting ground.
I explore what's lurking in my brain
And see if it is sound.

I like to read the comments
That I get online from others.
And if I want to get some more,
I call and get my mother's.

This therapy—it isn't cheap.
It costs a little time.
But the help that I've gotten,
Won't be forgotten.
I have a new paradigm!

I repeatedly realized that my tools were not much use to me unless I used them!

WHEN ALL ELSE FAILS
December 14, 2012

Some people finish this phrase with "read the instructions." But I'm thinking, "When all else fails, use the tools."

I used to collect diet books. *Fit Not Fat at Forty-Plus. Body Clutter. Perfect Weight. Why Can't I Stop Eating? The Four-Day Win.* There is something rather uncomfortable about staying obese with these books collecting dust on the shelves. And that's what was happening. Sure, the books looked promising, and they probably had a lot of good stuff in them. I even read some, but I wasn't following the instructions or using them as tools.

Even *Potatoes Not Prozac* sat on the shelf for a while after I bought it for a quarter at the used book sale. I had read enough on the back cover to think it might provide an answer for me. But I also had read enough to not want that answer to be my ticket to good health. Cutting out sugar? Keeping a journal of foods and moods? No eating between meals? There was a period of denial. And then anger. And then acceptance. Implementation. And, finally, thankfulness.

Potatoes Not Prozac shed some light on why I could lose weight but could never keep it off. It gave me some instruction on how to gain control over my eating. But it wasn't until I started *using* the directions that I lost my cravings for sweets.

I already knew WW was a good program. But it wasn't until I started *using* the tools effectively along with my sugar-addiction awareness that it really worked for me.

I just had an annual physical this morning. My doctor was very pleased with how far I've come with my health in the last year. My cardiology testing this past summer showed that my heart could handle exercise very well. I'm in excellent shape for a fifty-year-old!

This post brewed in my mind for quite some time. It's not about coffee. It is about meekness.

POINT OF CONTROL
December 15, 2012

Meekness isn't weakness
But rather strength under control
And the place this has the most meaning
Is how it pertains to my soul.

But this blog is about my weight loss
And that's what I'll talk about.

The things I have proven along the way
Of which I have not a doubt.

I've talked about what sugar does
To my brain and how I eat.
I've talked about starting diets strong
And then beating a hasty retreat.

Back to the land of sugar in control
Not eating in public but hidden.
Packing on the weight again
Miserable and guilt ridden.

And then the light in my head went on
When I came across a book.
Potatoes Not Prozac offered a chance
And it was, finally, one I took.

I first resented following the plan
I thought I could do it myself.
I thought I was smart and strong enough willed
And the book spent some time on the shelf.

But then I saw that I really couldn't
Do this thing on my own.
I had tried it time and time again
And successes always got blown.

So I picked up the book and submitted
To the author's research and advice
And once I got rid of the sugar
I found things were rather nice.

Sugar had messed with my impulse controls
And freedom from that was amazing.
When I meekly accepted I needed some help,
Cut out sugar, and stopped all the grazing!

I could use my strength more effectively
When I had this new control.
Adding the use of the WW tools
Helped lead to my healthy weight goal!

And now as I work
On sustaining success
I'll stay in control
With a little meekness.

I had to work on handling things with care.

TACTILE
December 21, 2012

I didn't see that one coming. I just felt it this morning and decided to see where it would go. I was thinking that this whole weight-loss and healthy-living deal is a hands-on thing. Keeping in touch with how I feel inside can help me keep my hands off foods I shouldn't put inside me.

I physically gather ingredients to prepare meals in a healthy way. Yesterday I was at the grocery store and actually picked up a few items that I know I shouldn't eat. (Not the diet thing—the sugar addict thing.) I thought about how they would feel to eat. And then I thought about how I would feel after that. I put them back. And I got by a rough patch.

Yesterday was a strange day. I consumed a lot of food. And then I ate some more. I felt out of control. And then I realized that was a mirror of how I felt about a couple of other situations in my life right now.

I may have sounded in control in my blog posts, but sometimes I have trouble after writing. The fat monster inside stirs and says, "Do you *really* think that?" And, "Have you *really* changed your paradigm?" And, "You may look thin on the outside, but I'm feeling like you *really* are fat."

I was glad when yesterday was over. And I was nervous this morning that it could set up to be a similar day. But I had a place where I could leave the things I can't control. And with *tact*, *I'll* say to myself today, "There are things you *can't* control, but what you eat is not one of them."

Out-of-control eating doesn't make the things I can't control any better. It just makes me feel worse. I need to keep the tools in my hands. And even if I can't see quite clearly, they'll help me feel my way along in the right direction. Reduced sugar. Drinking instead of eating between meals. Tracking. Taking a multivitamin. It works. It's worth doing. That's the point. And it feels good.

I looked at words and then looked at them again. I often found little things inside them that made me … think!

THiNK
December 23, 2012

It's rather obvious there's a *thin* inside of *think*. And for me to be thin and to stay thin (because I think I need to remember that I *am* thin right now), I need to think. Thin oKay!

There's a good chance I won't get to write for the next week or so. But I can still ThinK. And that's the plan. I know avoiding sugar will help me ThinK clearly. Avoiding between-meal eating will help me too. I will thinK about having enough water, a daily vitamin, and omega-3s. I'll work on getting vitamin D in sunshine or liquid form. I'll exercise by hauling gear, skiing, and smiling.

This next post is the reality of a slipup while I was on vacation.

MiND OVER MADDER
December 28, 2012

This thought came to me this morning. The better-known phrase is mind over matter, but I was getting madder and madder over not sticking with my plan. I was eating as if I didn't mind the consequences. And I attribute it to just a little sugar at a time. Just a little grazing between meals that snowballed into an avalanchical freefall everywhere except for the scale.

So this morning, I'm minding instead of getting madder. Mind over madder. The past few days have been justavacation, and they are over. That is settled in my mind, and now I'm not madder.

I went to an early exercise class this morning. I was a little nervous because I had some problems with my new ski boots this week and my toes were affected, but I went. I was able to do everything with gusto and feel good about it.

I'm coming up to my one-year anniversary of online working the tools for real. I could focus on the fact that I was two-tenths of a pound away from my seventy-five-pound star a few weeks ago and that I'm more than that now. Or I could focus on the fact that I am still here.

This journey has been more about my mind than my weight loss. Although the weight loss was important and needed, my mind needed help. Sure, I've had a slipup or two. But I also had a slip down a week or so ago (my slip was too big and started slipping down). I have not given up. That matters big time in a smaller body with a clearer mind.

There is a big possibility I will have a headache from sugar and refined carb withdrawal, but it will be worth it. I don't think I'll mind it so much, because it's better to have that than to have madder. Madder at myself for caving. Madder at myself for being human. (And what good does that do? I *am* human. I try to have great patience with others who are working at this process, and it's appropriate for me to have at least a little patience with myself!)

To take this a little further, I will mind the consequences of choices. I will pay attention before I make the choice. I have proved to myself that I am sensitive to sugar. There is something about it that messes with my impulse control over food and other things. It's what has derailed my previous attempts to lose weight by making me not mind (or care) about being heavy in the moment of eating and eating and eating some more. I could be the perfect "dieter" for a day or a week or a month and then wreck it in a fifteen-minute feeding (sugar) frenzy from which I would take months or seasons or years to recover.

Sugar isn't easy to avoid, bit I've proven it can be done. Because it matters. To my body and my mind. And so, with this information and the WW online tracking tools and community, I've been working to change my mind. The way I think about food (logging points). The way I move (exercise tracking). The way I process what is happening in my experience with the tools (blogging). Losing and learning to live at a healthy weight. It's not a diet; it's a paradigm with a positive spin. For the most part, it's a happy thing.

Yes. I choose mind over madder!

The idea of writing about a popular Christmas plant came into my mind out of season, but I saved the thought until the timing was right. Perhaps that's why it came out in a poem.

POINSETTIA (SEASONAL ADJUSTMENT)

December 30, 2012

Last week, this gal who tracks points

Etta lot—till she felt out of joint.
She stopped in mid choke—
But not up in smoke—
The bridge to good health was not boint.

I'd say that it was in the Nick o' time
The brakes went on to straighten my spine
The sudden jolt:
"Drop the nuts and bolt!"
Don't eat some more—just go rhyme!

So back to my tools and this train of thought
I'll track what I chew-chew and do what I ought.
If I'm up on the scale
There's no need to wail.
I'll hit target when I aim my best shot!

Other times, I'd pick a topic and run with it whether I had the ball or not.

GOAL POST
December 31, 2012

I don't know much about football. But I know about tracking. Well, food tracking anyway. Not big- or small-game tracking. Life tracking. Not so much fast tracking. Enough. Well, actually, that's the problem. I haven't been doing it enough.

I guess this is a big time for football. In the fringes of my mind, I know there are college bowls being played. Well, they're not playing in the fringes of my mind. But it's happening somewhere. The Super Bowl is coming up. I know about that from the grocery store circulars every year.

Speaking of circulars, this revolution around the sun is coming full circle pretty soon. It's a time of resolutions and goal setting. And it's a time of reflection. It's also a time for parties.

Maybe there *is* a football game going on in my mind. There seems to be a bit of passing going on. A few interceptions. I don't know if I got ten yards in the first four attempts at paragraphs. I think there's something related to that in the sports game. I do know I have some things I need to tackle.

I need to get my *Potatoes Not Prozac* book back, or get a new one. I got the first copy for a quarter. I don't want my quarter back. I just need the book back! I want to refresh my memory. I want to see the goal clearer. I know it's close. And I don't want to lose more ground before I see it again.

I'm writing this in a bit of a sugar haze. I haven't been successful at breaking it for more than a day and a half since my recent ski trip. I know I need four solid days of commitment to tracking, greatly reduced sugar, awareness, and no grazing between meals. Perhaps just writing this, posting it, and then going back and reading it in a few hours or so will let me see how wacky things are in my head.

I'm going to celebrate one year of online WW in two days. Clean. That's the goal. And this is the post.

And so the first year ended, and the next one started. More of the same. I was still working on changing my mind.

KNiFEPOiNT
January 7, 2013

Maybe it's more like the cutting edge. I try to keep my wits sharp so my posts won't be dull. For lunch on Sunday, I had planned to make a chopped salad, baked chicken breast, and oven "fried" potato wedges (French fries). The original plan was for my husband, daughter, and me. But at the last minute, we had company, and I wasn't comfortable with how much chicken I'd baked. (There's comfort food, and then there's the comfort of having enough food.) There was a slight problem with the potatoes. Instead of French fries, we had petrified potatoes because I left them in the oven too long.

I went shopping in my deep freeze and found a two-pound bag of shrimp. My pantry had whole-wheat thin spaghetti. While I was bringing the water to boil for the pasta, I started thawing and shelling the shrimp. Then, with my knife, I turned the leftover veggie sticks (carrots, celery, snap peas, and red peppers) from Saturday's lunch into stir-fry (with a little sesame oil, soy sauce, garlic, red onion, and powdered ginger). The pasta and shrimp got boiled (separately). I sliced up and plated the chicken. (I knew some folks didn't care for shrimp.) And when I brought it all to the table, we had the makings of do-it-yourself lo mein with sriracha sauce and homemade hot-pepper jam for condiments. Oh, I also threw together a simple tossed salad while I was fixing the other stuff. We had tea and yellow honeydew melon slices for dessert.

It sounds like a great day. And it pretty much was up to a point. And then I fell apart. I won't go into the details, because sometimes I think I have trouble writing and reading that information. Power of suggestion and all that. It has been tracked and the quantity is too. Much, that is.

We were invited to a late-afternoon get-together that involved finger foods. And my original plan of veggie sticks and hummus disappeared with lunch. So I made some sweets and some scones.

I'm giving this a lot of thought. And I'm thinking some of my rebelliousness and reckless abandon might have something to do with my reaction to my experience at the WW career fair I went to on Saturday.

I feel like I'm on the cutting edge of self-discovery. And that's a major victory in the making. No one and nothing is being held or made to do anything at knifepoint. I think what's going to shake out from this is some downsizing in my attitude, which will help me keep my downsized clothing. I also have fresh reassurance of my personal need to lay off sugar, no matter what anyone says about it. I have to cut out some illogical thinking. I'll leave it to cleaver. Cut it now and not wait for June.

Life isn't perfect. Sometimes circumstances change, and I have to scramble. But I'm learning to use what I have. Guidelines and tracking tools to fit each situation. Before, during, or after disaster. Or maybe, sometimes, averting disaster. Always learning. In each experience. Right through lifetime.

SUGARHOLIC OR NOT

Finding Enough Proof

When I reactivated my free lifetime status with WW, I opted to go to the weekly meetings. I guess I wanted to see if I had conquered whatever hang-ups I had from previous attempts with WW meetings. I met people and had lots of opportunities to share my success story. My leader asked me to participate in a One Amazing Day event at the center. I would be a guest speaker in the morning and afternoon sessions of a company-wide open house. My leader also asked me if I'd attend a career fair to see if I might like to work for WW. All of this was flattering and exciting, but there was a downside that I wasn't prepared for.

REACTIONS
January 7, 2013

I like what I've been doing over the past year. But in order to stay on track, there is more work I need to do with my reactions to certain situations. I have to be accountable to myself. Not to the WW center or receptionist or leader. They are there for support not for policing. It is a resource but not a place of judgment.

Last Saturday, I went to a WW career fair not really knowing what to expect. My former leader had asked me if I had considered working for WW. I decided to see what the possibilities were. Everyone there was very friendly and very excited about working for WW. Everyone there had a history losing and maintaining healthy weight. Some had lost weight in a fairly short amount of time, and one lady had taken fifteen years to reach her healthy weight. They were all real people.

The format was more like visiting than interviewing. The setup was to try out the spaces of receptionist, product sales, and meeting leader. I was a little concerned about the product sales because some of the items were things I actually abused under the guise of, "Oh, it must be good for me. It's a WW product." It wasn't a reflection on WW exactly, but it was because I didn't know what sugar was doing to my brain and impulse controls. So I said something about encouraging people to use products that were helpful in supporting their weight-loss efforts. I also wondered out loud if, for me, trying to sell some of that stuff would be akin to an alcoholic being a bartender. But the support thing was the key idea, and she picked up on that.

I had a question about an upcoming event where I had been asked to share my story. And my former leader came over to talk with me. She requested that I not talk too much about sugar when I presented my success story at the One Amazing Day event the following week. I said I didn't think it was everyone's problem and that I wouldn't suggest that it was the answer for everyone. It was and still is, however, a big factor in my success. I thanked her, said I'd let her know what I thought about the career fair, and headed home.

I should have been excited when I left the career fair. But for some reason, I felt sad, confused, and disappointed that I was being asked to modify my story. I understood that the leader was just protecting the sales pitch of WW that nothing was off limits in their program. But I knew that I, personally, had to work with my guidelines for sugar management in order to keep my success story a success. I think a better request would have been to ask me to talk about individuals personalizing their use of the WW options and tools for success.

In the process of being requested to downplay the sugar aspect of my story, a little thought started a wedge of wonder. Is it really that big of a deal for me to stay away from sugar and not eat between meals? I was telling an uncle about this later and he said, "That sounds like an alcoholic."

I'm going to pay attention to *my* success story. And I'm going to remember that it's mine. My success story began with realizing I'm sensitive to sugar. WW is part of my story, because I use their tracking tools and participate in their blogging community.

Re: Action. I'm working it.

My experience with the meeting format really reinforced my appreciation of the support I felt in the WW online blogging community. I liked that 24/7 access to support and encouragement while also supporting and encouraging others. Here's my real reaction!

HOME ON THE BLOGS
January 7, 2013

Oh give me a home, where the WW roam,
And the blogs and the boards work all day.
Where seldom is read a discouraging thread
And reading keeps hunger at bay.

Home, home on the range
Where I cook low-point chicken satay.
Where nothing is burned; it's a new lesson learned
And I'm working t'ward good health today.

How often I write, when I have a new plight
With the light from my computer screen.
I've sat here amazed, and smiled slightly dazed—
My friends really get what I mean!

Home, home on the blogs!
Where the WW write night and day.
Where answers are found that help and astound
And inspire me to point out my way!

I might take a stand. Say no food that is bland
Or have slightest resemblance to diet.
I'm working the tools with my personal rules
And checking on folks that are quiet.

Oh I would not exchange and it's not all that strange
When I think of the pounds that I've lost.
I've gained lots of friends, on their blogs I depends
Gently guided and not loudly bossed.

Home, home on the blogs!
Where the WW write night and day.
Some posts are absurd, most encouraging words
To help me in losing my weigh(t).

Thanks to Dr. Brewster M. Higley (1823–1911) for the original lyrics.

There are a lot of posts from this time period. Some seem silly, but they're all a part of me hanging on to control. Part of my strategy was to type instead of eating between meals. I know I could have snacked my way through to a complete derailment of tracking, but I didn't. I typed and typed and typed some more.

TiME TO NOTiCE SOME NON-SCALE ViCTORiES
January 8, 2013

I've been stuck in a rut
Of reas'ning and "but"
When I really should focus on more:
E'en the things that are right
(like my clothes—not too tight)
Instead of becoming a bore!

(As an aside,
And not to be snide
A boar is a type of wild pig.
When sugar hogs my focus
There's a certain hocus-pocus
That's conducive to flipping my wig.)

My original title
To this little writel
Was "Time for an NSV."
But on further thought
It was clear that I ought
To just *notice* and really see!

I just tripped and stumbled
And got a bit jumbled
But didn't get too far off track.
I kept on moving
(Though out of my grooving)
And went yakkity-yakkity-yack.

Now it is clear
The tools I hold dear
Are an NSV just in the using.
There's a short time to pout
I did that, no doubt,
And then spent some time on the musing.

Here is another
For me and my brother

(if I had one,) or p'rhaps for my sister.
I seek out support
For a pleasant retort
Or perhaps a kick in the keister!

I'm using the tools!
I see them as jewels!
To display in an empowered crown!
There's so much to cheer!
I'm healthy and here!
My smile is up! And my weight will get down!

I continued to struggle with my thoughts about my story. And so I continued to write about it!

A FEW MORE THOUGHTS ON NSV
January 9, 2013

I posted in my status yesterday: NSVs Non-Scale Victories or **Need Some Validation** or maybe both.

That gave me cause
To pause
To stroke my jaws
Consider laws
And perhaps some flaws.
Yeah. I thought about it more.

This whole deal of weight loss dwells a lot on the negative. At the scale anyway. It's a positive thing when the number is negative. And when the change is positive, the feeling is negative. Enter the non-scale victory. It's basically recognition of positive things that don't show up at the scale. Clothes fitting better, meeting a challenge, getting a compliment from someone, being happy about using the tools, noticing new things to be thankful for—lots of different things.

The new thought was about Need Some Validation. I need to recognize that my journey is important. My story is *my* success story. I need to understand that how I choose to use the WW tools (resources) is valid for *me*. As in: blogging my way through struggles. Coming out on the other side to write a goofy but thought-provoking rhyme. Exercising before blogging. As in: it works for me.

In writing and reading my thoughts, there's a certain level of validation (establishing soundness). I suppose it's even more so (sound) if I read it out loud! The comments I get reinforce that (or tell me I'm certifiable!). And I'm thankful for the feedback. (I am so thankful for feedback that I also try to comment on several blogs a day!)

Why doubts creep in is a mystery. Unless one considers the human mind. That can explain a lot. It's still a mystery, but it's okay. Perhaps it's one of those laws of nature. There is a lot of "wiring" and electricity in our brains, but they don't all work the same way. We're not robots. External and internal situations have an impact. And sometimes just recognizing them and noticing they exist can help.

Last Friday my WW leader talked about hedonic eating. She asked us how we felt about hormones and cravings and what they can make us do. (Eat when we're not hungry. Eat for the pleasure of it.) I said I thought it was empowering information because knowing why there's a problem can lead to a solution. (And we know the New Year is a great time for re:solutions.) It has to do with awareness.

I've lost a lot of weight. And I've had a lot of people ask me how I did it. I've talked about my sugar addiction. And had a feeling of being dismissed. Even by my doctor. When I talk about blogging, I get the same feeling. As if it's not a valid method of weight loss. When I talk about using the WW tools, there's some recognition of a valid method. But sometimes I feel I've been cubbyholed into a diet. It shouldn't matter to me. But it does. Because when I've used WW as a diet, it *hasn't* worked for me.

I use the online tools in conjunction with what I've learned about my body and my needs. This has provided me with Nice Scale Victories and Non-Scale Victories. When I Need Some Validation I get it. (And I don't feel like I Need Some Valium.)

The One Amazing Day event was on January 12, 2013. I bought a new outfit, gave my talks, answered questions, and felt anxious about the sugar part of my story. In reading over the next few blogs, I realized that I had some things to overcome regarding my addiction. My blog posts were doing exactly what I needed them to do. They kept me actively thinking about what was going on.

A.W.A.R.E.

January 15, 2013

When I was preparing for my One Amazing Day talk, my husband suggested I write some key points on note cards. One of the cards said "Awareness."

I can't remember the other specific words right now, but I remember that as I practiced talking about my success, it seemed like every point I made was circling back to awareness.

A key awareness for me was reading the book *Potatoes Not Prozac*. I was aware that I had a problem that was supporting my obesity. This book helped me see what the problem was and how I could change my approach to food so I would be in control—and not the food in control of me. I joined WW online to use the tracking tools and found a few other tools that have helped me in my journey to a healthy weight.

Tracking is a tool of awareness.
Blogging is a tool of awareness.
The scale is a tool of awareness.
A tape measure is a tool of awareness.
Measuring cups are tools of awareness.
Appreciate **W**hat **A**wareness **R**eally **E**nables.

Awareness has helped me recognize I have choices and consequences. If I choose to eat sugar and graze between meals, I am choosing to live in a sugar-hazed fog that makes me feel out of control, ashamed, and guilty.

If I choose to eat much less sugar and keep my eating to mealtimes with start and stop times, I am choosing to be in control of my health with better mental clarity and more-even moods.

I could go on and on. But I have to stop here, because I chose to go skiing today (good) and also chose to disregard my eating guidelines (not so good). I'm feeling rather glad that I'm feeling rather bad. I think I had gotten too far away from the memory of my initial sugar detox.

Awareness. A little more awareness would have enabled me to be aware of my need of hydrating instead of carbohydrating! A little more awareness would have had me drinking fluids until mealtime, even if it meant visiting the ladies' room more often. I'm not feeling sorry for myself. I'm being aware. And that's going to involve thankfulness. I'm not beating myself up. I would have in the past, but I'm aware that practicing self-bashing for something like this leads to a downward spiral in mood, not scale. I'm just being A.W.A.R.E. **A**lways **W**orking **A** **R**esponsible **E**xplanation.

As I continued to struggle, I continued to work the thoughts in my mind. I know that I got a bit weary of slipups and trying to regain control. But if I had just given up, it would have been a terrible waist (pun intended).

BRAKE VS. BREAK
January 18, 2013

A few people are aware of my recent struggles with sugar. I am more convinced than ever before that I am addicted to sugar. It can be in a piece of candy, a piece of fruit, processed foods, or whole grains. It doesn't always show up right away, but the little things chip away and then *pow*! I am out of control.

A reader might think, "Enough already!" Just cut the stuff out and quit writing about it. But that's not the point. Although I *know* that I have a problem with sugar, I'm still *learning* how to balance my brain. And just as a toddler doesn't get chewed out for falling when learning to walk, I don't need to have expectations of perfect as I'm learning to balance. What I'm needing is an early warning system so I can put the *brakes* on before I *break*. I've come up with some acronyms!

Be **R**eal **A**nd **K**now **E**verything. That translates to log and blog. I've had some days when I've not wanted to blog. I've felt guilty and ashamed of my slipups. I've felt like a fraud. My husband was a big encouragement to me this morning when he told me that my accomplishment is real, and there is nothing fraudulent about it even if I'm struggling right now.

If that BRAKE seems a bit harsh, I also have **B**alance **R**easonable, **A**ppropriate, **K**ind **E**xpectations.

Last night I felt like I was ready to BREAK. **B**inge **R**eact **E**at **A**nd **K**ick. (Me on too much sugar.) I'd had a day and a half of clean. And then my plans got rearranged. I ordered something that didn't turn out to be what I thought it was. The fried onions weren't pan fried, they were "can fried." Although I used just a little of the dressing that was on the side, it had too much sugar in it. Better planning could have prevented this. But it happened. Later on, I caught myself looking for an excuse to go out and get "drunk" or "high" on a hot fudge sundae or several candy bars or even a Big Mac. Fortunately, that didn't happen. But the thought was there. I knew the dragon was awake.

I have a few stressors going on right now, but that is part of life. There are a few situations I am very aware of that I would like to help take care of. But I can't. I have absolutely no control or say in how things go. And I have to accept that no matter how they turn out, I am not responsible for the outcome. What I also need to accept is that *none of that is a reason for me to fall apart with sugar.*

Back to the sugar thing. It affects my mood in a terrible way. I lose my spark and ready smile. I don't feel like me. I have to get going with other things right now But I've just come up with another way to stop, or brake, the sugar thing. It's big.

Blog Review And Keep Exercising. That's it.

I would think I had things under control, and then I'd go into a spin again. And a gain. The touch of humor showed me I was still in there.

DiSGRUNTLED
January 21, 2013

I started to spin out of control with sugar-related eating again. And just before I caught myself, I was eating like a pig! I won't go into details. I'll just say I'm glad we didn't go to any all-you-can-eat feeding-trough restaurants while I was under the influence of sugar!

Detox, the first time, was physically painful with a severe headache and feeling miserable from cold-turkey quitting sugar. This time, and I think it's because of my increased physical activity, the reaction to detox is more in how I'm feeling emotionally.

I noticed a few times of anxiety and other times of grumpiness. But with my heightened awareness, I recognized it could just be from sugar detox. That recognition saved me from a downward spiral of emotional eating. I increased my intake of omega-3 and held on to my guidelines for managing sugar addiction. I've come through it. And on the other side was a clarity and calmness that I crave more than sugar.

I'm on day three of clean eating. I can't relax with regard to this sugar thing. But I'll feel more comfortable with four days of clean eating and then five and then six and on and on and on.

I've proved to myself a few times that this is serious. And I have proven a few times that I can rein myself in. Not by dieting, but by doing what works.

It's so nice to not be oinking anymore. I'm disgruntled!

Having slipups with sugar and then working to regain control could be a downer. But I tried, and succeeded more times than not, to find a happy place.

HAPPY NEW WEEK!
January 22, 2013

I battled the dragon, Sugar.
It put up a mighty strong fight.
But I finally got my head on straight
And I feel like things are now right.

Not very far into last week,
I found I was eating too much.
Not just too much but in between meals—
With my needs, I was out of touch.

I had wakened the dragon, Sugar,
(doesn't it sound so sweet?)
Played with fire and got a bit scorched
By choosing the wrong things to eat.

Historically, or hysterically,
This would have been the demise
Of all the progress I'd made last year
And my weight would be quick on the rise.

I wrote my way through—with some help from friends
And I'm oh so thankful for this!
I'm still on track and am able to yack
And I'm feeling like nothing's amiss.

Well, some weight has gone missing,
But that I'm not dissing.
It's a result of doing what works.
I'm using the tools with my PNP rules.
I'm aware of the dragon that lurks!

Part of that dragon is sugar
And part of its nature is diet.
When I focus on health and not on the scales
I win! And I urge folks to try it!

So back to the title
Of this, my post:
Happy New Week
Make it your boast!

Now for a little more about this past week, because thinking about it was helpful to me. Even though I felt completely out of control early in the week, I was with it enough to keep tracking even if it wasn't completely accurate. Perhaps it would have been better to itemize every detail. But that's not the point at this time. The point is that *every single morning*, I had potential for a Happy New Day. I had hope. And it worked. I didn't have to wait for a new week to recover.

And when I weighed myself this morning on my scale at home, I was down five pounds. I've lost that five pounds a few times in the past two months. *But this time I feel really good about it. Because it was a side effect of working the tools that work for me.* Living in good health. Not on a diet.

I will weigh in at the WW center later this week when I go to a meeting. That will be for WW and to maintain my free eTools. But I've decided I need to keep my official weigh-in for me, and my health, at home. Because that works for me.

Though I thought I would miss my sugar,
I don't miss how it made me behave.
I'm finding more and more these days,
It's health and control I crave!

In all of life's challenges, it is easy to lose focus on some points that are worth remembering.

REMEMBERING THE POINT

January 25, 2013

I've had some challenges this week. But staying on plan has not been one of them. Staying on plan has actually been a comfort to me.

Last Friday I went to my WW meeting and didn't weigh in. It was a scary place for me to be. I didn't *have* to weigh in, but I have weighed in every other time I've been there since reinstating my lifetime status. I stayed for the meeting. I tried to soak in some good vibes, and then I went to the grocery store where I acted like someone trying to beat the system. I acted like I used to act when I was *on* WW and not *using* WW. I inhaled a bag of day-old pastries in a very short amount of time. And that wasn't all. Oh no. That was not all. But that's all I'm going to write about.

I worked through some issues by blogging. I knew I was out of control, and I knew why. I just didn't seem to be able to care enough until I had done considerable damage on my tracker. I had gone in and out of the red zone already that week. And maybe it took a second bunch of red to jolt me to my senses and make me ask myself if I really wanted to have to get rid of my thin clothes again after stretching them out like sausage skins.

Some of my struggle came through in my writing. And I had some online friends checking in on me. Some offered support, and some offered a bit of a lecture! When my husband quietly asked me, with no judgment attached, "Are you having trouble with sugar?" the resistance to accepting help and helping myself melted away, and I was relieved to get back to what had worked so well over the past fourteen months.

I recommitted to tracking and no grazing between meals. Enough protein. Reduced sugar. Vitamin every day. Exercise. Clean eating. I've strung a few days together. I've read and commented on blogs. And in trying to encourage others, I have encouraged myself.

I'm feeling safer with the comfort of tracking. And that is the point.

It takes some commitment to stick with a plan in sickness and in health. I got sick, but not too sick to rhyme.

ODE TO A RETCH-ED DAY
January 29, 2013

This retch-ed day has been pointing the way
To my bathroom with bucket in hand.
I've not eaten a thing but tucked head under wing
And not thought about food, even bland.

I think that the tide is now turning
My body is glad that it's time.

How, you may ask, do I know I'll get better?
Well, I'm starting to think in a rhyme.

My head it has been pounding
In my eyes and down to my jaws.
But I'm able to drink some clear liquids
And my temp doesn't spark arctic thaws.

Well, I really don't know how high my temp went
But it worked with the words in that stanza.
Poetic license can do that sometimes
And I take it for a bonanza.

There's something refreshing about not eating food
Though it's not often been my habit.
I'm working a cleansing quicker than fast—
Opportunity with no choice but to grab it.

Yes, I feel miserable and that's how it goes
When the stomach bug makes an appearance.
But I looked for and found a positive side
That will help me with my endurance.

Though this little bug has made a big splash
It's not much more than a pain.
I'm glad of wishes for me getting better—
I'll soon be back on the train.

Even in sickness there were lessons to observe.

BACK ON THE TRAIN
January 30, 2013

There haven't been many days in my life where I haven't had any food
at all. Yesterday was one. And now that's done. Or at least I hope it is.
I finally felt like eating food this morning. I heated up some brown rice,
poached a couple of eggs (fresh from my friend's chickens), and had a
banana. Once I started eating, I felt really hungry. But I couldn't finish
everything on my plate, which is fine. I'm not interested in piling too
much on to begin with, but I think I'm interested in leaving a little left
over. Just to see what it's like. And to pay attention to how I'm feeling—
not what I'm seeing.

On Monday I was eating for something else. On Tuesday I wasn't eating at all. (I suppose it could be called reverse eating.) Today I am eating to feed my body. So far, so good.

The battle with scale numbers couldn't take away the victories off the scale.

NON-SCALE VICTORIES TO NOTICE
January 31, 2013

I am here.

I am not just starting.

And I'm not just finishing up.

I'm in my healthy-weight range.

I've been in my healthy weight range since August 2012.

I haven't lost sight of reaching my healthy "heart" weight whatever that happens to be.

I'm proving to myself that I have what it takes to maintain.

I've proved to myself that I have what it takes to blow up like someone pulled the pin on an inflatable life raft. Except it wouldn't be a life raft, it would be the means of me sinking into despair and rising on my weight tracker.

But I digress.

The WW tools work for me when I pay attention to my sugar-management plan.

My clothes are not tight on me.

Clothes that I used to think were my skinny clothes are too big.

I never thought I would wear a size small again. And then I tried on my daughter's extra-small, tall workout pants. They fit me.

I feel good about a lot of things when I'm eating clean.

Tracking isn't a weight-loss tool. It's an awareness tool.

The scale is not my enemy. It helps me be aware of where I am and what I can wear.

Blogging is a true life raft when I get in over my head.

Which reminds me of a quote I once read, "If you're in over your head, keep your mouth shut."

I can keep my mouth shut and refrain from eating through my emotions. And I can use my fingers with a keyboard to keep my mind open to possibilities and solutions. More awareness stuff.

I have run over seven miles in eighty minutes. For fun.

My husband likes to run with me.

My quads don't kill me when I ski.

I have an amazing support system with the online community. Friends I've never met (most of them, anyway) but truly care for.

Yeah.

I have a lot of things for which to be thankful.

I think it was a relief to me when January was over. But I wasn't letting down my guard.

FIB, YOU'RE WARY
February 1, 2013

This thought came to me last night when I was thinking about January 2013 sliding into history. January is historically a month to start diets. And I found partway through the month that I was in diet mode. It was messing me up by getting in my head and crowding out the reasonableness of just using the tools the way they work for me. The way to my success was to be honest with myself.

I love the signature of one of my friends—she makes a comment about the body always tracking with perfect accuracy. So why wouldn't I embrace truth in tracking if I wanted to really see what was going on with my eating habits?!

Truth in tracking leads to peace of mind. When you fib, you're wary. I think February could be considered a month when many people quit diets or healthy eating plans. Less than truthful and a bit wary of what's going on at the scale. The tools don't work if they're not used.

I'm going to use this little play on words to raise my awareness level. Truth in tracking. Next month could be all about activity. (March!)

And then there were boot-i-full days!

BOOTS AND REBOOTS
February 11, 2013

It is boot weather, and we have a ton of snow to make tracks in. I've decided it's also reboot season for me. And tomorrow's start of a new week has plenty of room for fresh tracks.

I was talking to a friend today. She's someone who first met me at my very heaviest weight a few years ago. She commented that she really doesn't notice me as having lost a lot of weight. She says I just seem like me. That may not make a lot of sense to everyone, but it made lots of sense to me. I'm glad she said it.

It has been holiday season. And winter doldrums season. And whatever the reason, I'm still hanging out at the higher end of my healthy-weight range. I've noticed my wrists are really small, and that's telling me that I really don't belong in the large-frame category. I feel like a shaky success story.

So I'm going to reboot. Tomorrow's weigh-in will be my new starting weight. I'm going to use my online tools in conjunction with the guidelines I follow from *Potatoes Not Prozac*. I'm going to revisit the book (I have a copy again) and start from the back section—the part I never really read.

I'm going to keep my weigh-in day on Tuesday at home. I may or may not go to the meetings for a while. I'm just going to do what worked last year. Log, jog, and blog. Mini goals. Point-blank range. Can't miss. A little reboot kick in the right place helps!

Speaking of boots, I really like my new boots. They are a regular size, and they are not in the least bit tight on my calves. I don't feel like a cow in them even though they are leather!

One of the first chapter books I listened to (other than the Bible) was Charlotte's Web. *My mom read it to my older sister not knowing if I was taking any of it in until I burst into tears when Charlotte died. I've read the book on my own several times since then. There are life lessons that still work today.*

WRITING ON THE WEB
February 12, 2013

Last year at this time, I was blissfully blogging my way through munchies. I was reading blogs and commenting on them. I was writing posts to my blog and starting to get comments on them. I was drinking Good Earth Sweet and Spicy Tea or seltzer or just plain water when I thought I was hungry between meals. I was tracking truer than a bloodhound. I was working my tools, and they were working for me.

This year at this time, I'm writing in my blog instead of grazing through the late afternoon and evening. Yesterday I wasn't doing that. But that was yesterday. And yesterday is gone. I'm thinking about today. And tomorrow. And the next day. But mostly about today, because it's what I've got. Right now, I'm making good choices, and I'm feeling like it's worth it.

I was rereading my *Potatoes Not Prozac* book this afternoon while I was waiting for my daughter at the dentist office. And for all the writing I've done about this book, I was amazed with some of the things I came across.

Granted, this is a different edition from the one I originally purchased at the library book sale. But for some reason, I hadn't picked up on the last step and the feeling of being radiant. (As an aside, I think of Wilbur the pig in *Charlotte's Web* when I think of radiant. It's not so helpful for a weight-loss image, but I have fond memories of that book!)

I didn't remember reading about radiant, but I do remember living it. And I also remember not living it before I read the book and several occasions in recent months. The concept of radiant tells me that living clean and aware is more than my weight and the shape of body. It's also about my mind.

I read enough this afternoon to know that I want to read the beginning of *Potatoes Not Prozac* again. I read just enough of the first edition of the book in 2011 to feel validated in my feelings of being like an alcoholic with sugar. Once I started acting on the information, I lost a lot of weight as one of the side effects. The radiance was another side effect. I just didn't know what it was called.

Somewhere along the line I lost a little of that. I think it had to do with raising my goal weight to the high end of my range, so I could secure my free online tools and lifetime status again. I've been as low as my original lifetime goal weight (fifteen pounds lighter than my max) for a few minutes anyway but not officially. I also think I let some second-guessing creep in on my knowledge of what works. Sugar addiction is good at that.

I've bounced around enough lately to feel like I'm taking up the yo-yo game again. And I don't like it. A little too much leeway on the start and stop times to eating. A snitch here and there. A little sugar. A little and then a lot. Out of control and back. And forth. Not so radiant. And then a flash of light. A.W.A.R.E. **A**wareness **W**elcomes **A**lert **R**esponsible **E**ating. Or so it came to me this morning. The morning of my reboot action plan.

One of the things I read about this afternoon is awareness. The tracker is a tool of awareness. The blog is a tool of awareness. The scale is a tool of awareness. Reading blogs is a tool of awareness. (I'm not alone with struggles or noticing victories.) Commenting is a tool of awareness. And I'm welcoming that thought.

I've written about it before. I'm aware of that. And I'm also aware that it's helpful for me to repeat positive things to myself. I'm aware of the radiance, and it makes me feel thankful. I'm aware of what takes that away. And I'm thankful to know what to avoid. And also to know that I can get it back.

I'm aware that this is a public document, but I'm also aware that I have to write it for me. Because, as I've said before, it's part of my life raft. It's part of what keeps my head above water and well out of the feeding trough. Radiant. But not "some pig."

My inspirations for blog posts could come from anywhere and everywhere. I don't think much happened without me considering it a possible writing prompt.

BAD ATTITUDE VS. BEATITUDE
March 6, 2013

I've been having a little trouble with my attitude lately. It's mostly due to lack of sleep, I think. And possibly due to that, I've made some poor food choices. Or perhaps it's in reverse order.

The suffix "itude" signifies a noun of state. Yesterday morning I was in a terrible state. Not a comment on Connecticut—just a bad attitude. I went back to bed and slept until noon. It helped. I went for a walk with my husband, and that helped. And then I went for a run, which was also helpful. I got a little more sleep last night.

Thankfulness is returning. Lack of sleep was impairing my vision. I wasn't seeing the positives. My thoughts weren't feeding on the right things. And neither was my body. With an attitude of gratitude, I'm feeling much happier.

So with regard to food, my mind sees an EAT in Beatitude. And that next to a *B* makes me think: You are what you eat. Or what you feed on. There's a lot of food for thought!

"Call Me Maybe" was a wildly popular pop song by Carly Rae Jepsen. I think some of the words influenced this next post.

WHAT'S MY NUMBER?
March 21, 2013

I set my goal weight at the highest in my healthy range last October when I decided to reactivate my lifetime status with WW. It had been more than twenty years since the original goal weight had been set. I was over fifty. It was allowed.

Since October, I've bounced around with my number on the scale. There have been several things going on that have contributed to the bouncing. Some of it is lack of sleep. A bit of stress. My weakened condition (which seemed to be worst on weekends) has played into my problems with sugar and how it messes with my impulse controls.

One thing that triggered my attention to this being a more serious problem than I had realized was that I noticed I wasn't weighing myself every day. I know daily weighing isn't encouraged by WW. And I know some people feel really guilty if they weigh every day.

But I've found that knowing my number is important for me. I was still weighing in officially every week. But as I was fighting with my sugar addiction more, I was worrying about my number more. And it was turning into a diet mentality thing. That's something that I've proved many times does not work for me. In worrying about it, I was avoiding the scale. It may not make sense, but that's what was happening. That's the story of all my previous attempts to be at a healthy weight.

I realized this morning that I simply need to use the WW tools as a way to track my foods and moods. I need to stick to my sugar-management guidelines for eating (no grazing, greatly reduced sugar, enough protein, enough water, a multivitamin). If I do this, I don't have to worry about what my goal weight number is. I'll be there and live there. It's not about dieting. It's about living in a way that is healthy for me. Doing it.

Weighing myself every day is just what I do. It's my number. Call me crazy. Or maybe. It just is what works for me. It doesn't have to be a downer if it's up. Or an upper if it's down. It's a snapshot of reality that keeps me grounded. Doing what I need to do for me. It's not a worry. It's aware.

I feel like I just met myself!

Not only was my blog a record of how I was feeling, but I was noting the length of the winter of 2013 in Connecticut!

SNOW MATTER
March 22, 2013

This morning came with a dusting of snow—
Powdered sugary, fine.
That's the way this spring has sprung
And it does no good to whine.

Also arriving this morning—
A brand-new tracking slate.
Opportunity ready and waiting
For good choices on my plate!

It's not that yesterday was very bad.
It actually went very well.
But approaching the day with this attitude
Just seems to ring the right bell.

It's not the start of a boxing match.
It's brand-new day of life!
And working the plan how it works for me
Tends not to be full of strife!

The weather or not—I can't control.
It's not warm, but daylight is longer.
The whether or not of what I eat
Can make me weaker or stronger.

In spite of powdered sugar snow
My outlook is sunny and warm.
As long as the sugar is not in me
I don't think I'll come to much harm!

Weather or not, I blogged!

PREDICTED VS. REALITY
March 26, 2013

The weather prediction for this fine day
Flirts with the fifties —WoooWeee!
I'll hope for the best but take what I get
'Cause I know how predictions can be!

Hope for the best but take what I get—
Sounds like a meeting with scale!
That's what I did on this morning so fine
And I've nothing at all to bewail.

The snapshot in time this morning
Showed a loss of eight pounds point two.
A reflection of paying attention again
And doing what I must do.

I'm back in the land of 160s again
And feeling closer to home.
This week I will simply follow my plan
And probably write a poem.

My prediction of writing a poem was accurate!

HMMMM

March 28, 2013

I have a slightly
Runny nose.
(It's not at all
Like a garden hose.)
And I only can think
In poems and not prose.
If I went to the clinic
Do you suppose
They would
Diagnose
Me with
Acute rhymitis?

I'll never know
Since I don't plan to go.
I took some Claritin instead.
Yes, the nose thing
Is because *spring*
Has arrived and simply gone to my head!
The poems and the rhymes and the playing with words
Seems a part of my DNA.
I'll try to be good
And refrain when I should.
Say things in a serious way.
You'd not think this poem's about weight loss
But it's a part of my plan (not a diet).
I'm writing, not eating, my thoughts in a blog.
It might work for you if you try it!

I didn't just stay at home and write poems, though. I was living life, and sometimes that meant road trips to see my folks. Typically, they were two-hour trips. Sometimes they turned into a trip in my plan, and sometimes they caused a great fall. I wrote about it all, and I learned a few things along the way.

IN CONTROL
April 4, 2013

Today I made another trip to see my dad who has been in the hospital since Sunday. The first trip this week was a bit of a disaster for me. But because it woke me up to what was happening with my sugar addiction, I actually feel thankful for it.

Today's trip went much better. I packed a lunch of leftover soup and some cold asparagus spears. I had enough seltzer to drink. For supper, I went to Subway and got a turkey chopped salad with lots of veggies but no olives or cheese. I chose red wine vinegar and oregano for dressing. I didn't feel like there was quite enough protein, so I went to the grocery store to round out the meal with a packet of turkey and some mango chunks. It was the same grocery store I went to on Tuesday. But this time, I wasn't interested in leftover Easter candy and cookies and pastries. That was a lovely feeling of control!

On the drive home today, I needed a break. I stopped at Wendy's, used the restroom, and then got a plain baked potato. No butter. No sour cream. Just salt and pepper and delicious. Exactly the right thing to keep me going until I got home.

This feeling of control is good. It's worth a lot. And I want to appreciate it. Value it. Guard it. With my lifetime!

I don't think I was obsessing about my sugar addiction, but I was keenly aware of it. Ideas of how to keep in control would pop up in my mind, and I'd explore them by writing words. Lots of words.

THE AFTER WORD
April 5, 2013

There's a helpful thought about being aware and present right now. But I'm having to think about after right now. The after word. Is it regret, or is it a sense of victory? Is it frustration or a sense of control? Doing a little fast-forward from the moment gives me a little boost to my tenuous grip of control. I can't be bold and say I've got this. But I can reach into my past and get a glimpse of what the after will be if I take a certain direction.

I've lived many years in and out of the clutches of sugar. I've had regrets and negative self-talk. I've eaten out of control even when I wanted to stop. It's something to do with hypersensitive neurotransmitters or something. I don't really understand the science of it, but there's more and more information coming out about the effects of sugar on a brain. There's scientific research, books, and magazine articles. It's a big deal. I know a lot about it up close and personal.

I know what it's like to be in the grip of sugar addiction. And I know what it's like to be sober. I know the high sugar produces. And I know it goes away all too quickly. I know it comes back soon enough as more and more sugar is consumed. But it takes away mental clarity. It takes away my impulse controls. It takes away my sense of me and builds a wall of fat around it.

I had months and months of sugar sobriety, and then I got involved in diet mentality. I focused on numbers, not how I was feeling and acting. I was losing weight, but I was also gaining it. Back to the yo-yo. Back to the sugar addiction. Back to the struggle. Trying to beat the system, I guess. And it doesn't work for me that way.

I know what works. I've documented it many times before (words). And I'm thinking I've discovered another thing that can work for me. The after word. It just may keep me going for words!

Today I can go to my WW meeting and weigh in within my lifetime numbers. But I'm not going to pay so much attention to the number. I'll stay for the meeting and all the words. The thing I'll be paying attention to is how I feel after the words. I'll report back after words.

As promised, I wrote about the next day's weigh-in. I like remembering the feeling of victory in actually doing what I had previously fretted about.

APRIL WEIGH-IN
April 5, 2013

I was in the free range. I'm so glad I wasn't too chicken to go to the WW meeting today!

I allowed enough time to weigh in and then go to Subway where I had a turkey chopped salad with extra meat. I had time to enjoy the salad and get back to the WW center for the meeting.

This week's meeting went well. I felt in control even though I hadn't been earlier in the week. Goof-ups happen, but I did something about it. I didn't let it continue. I made adjustments.

My victory was that I had weighed in the first week of the month. I was there, and that was a big deal. Having my lunch after weigh-in was a good plan. There was something really nice about sitting through a WW meeting with a satisfied tummy!

I hadn't seen that leader for a month or so, but she remembered my name. And she said she'd read my blog. During the meeting, there was a scenario with donuts, and I referred to a blog post I wrote last year. "Just Donut." The leader made a point to comment about my blog and suggested people look up *Pointing the Way*. I thought that was nice! I really appreciated her support.

I'm feeling good this evening. I got through my WW meeting without psychological baggage. I'm simply satisfied with how I've worked the tools today. Yes! I feel good about this. I'm working the tools with my plan. I'm not trying to beat a system. This is for my good. And it feels good!

Life is about choices. And a lot of what we choose has to do with chews.

CHEWSDAY! ANOTHER WEEK BITES THE DUST
April 9, 2013

I was biting some dust this afternoon while I was clearing some brush in the yard. I had three and a half hours of yard work in before I knew it. I finished up just in time to shower and get ready for my exercise class! Woo-hoo! Activity galore! I'll put it in my tracker, and if I want, I can eat some more!

This morning I was on the downward trend again at my official home weigh-in. I've been gaining and losing here and there. Stress and tiredness have made their play. I sometimes feel out of control, but most of the time I don't. I'm not as worried about numbers. They're just a tool to help me see where I am. I'm not into the guilt-trip thing like I used to be. I've been working the tools for more than a year, and I've been in my healthy-weight range for eight months. I'm going to consider that a huge victory!

This week and last week worked well for me. I've realized I can't eat too many grains. I've been careful to get enough protein at every meal. I'm working at eating only at mealtimes. Drinking enough water. Taking a multivitamin. And exercising.

I haven't experienced my usual head-game problems from my monthly weigh-in and WW meeting. I'm not sure how that happened, but I'm glad. My leader talked about the whack-a-mole game that weight loss and maintenance resemble. You think you've gotten something beaten, and something else pops up. When you whack that down, the other thing may have popped up again. And we keep going.

The big thing I think I have to remember is that the whack-a-mole game can be fun. And there doesn't have to be a lot of difference with the weight thing. I actually have had fun with my journey, thanks to blogging! I'll keep at it and keep getting my payoff: monthly tickets for free eTools! (Not to mention healthy!)

I'm heading into a busy end of the week. I have a plan. And I know it works! I just have to use it. I chews to use it! If there's a deviation from the plan, I can deal with it in a sensible way. That's how it works!

As I read about another sugar detox, it was obvious to me I had another slipup. But it was also obvious to me that I still cared enough to stop the slipup. As I've mentioned before, it's not a case of fixing my sugar addiction, but learning to live with it in a healthy way. The idea is to have clean eating be my new normal instead of the anomaly it was when sugar was in control.

MOVING RIGHT ALONG
April 18, 2013

I'm in day three of my sugar detox. And other than a twinge of a headache last night, I am feeling good. I have a feeling that being in better physical shape and having a written memory of what being free from sugar means for me is helping.

I enjoyed a walk with a friend this morning. She stopped by on her way to work, and we went about a mile together. We walk and talk. It's good for both of us. I have an exercise class to go to tonight. I don't have to go, but I want to go because I enjoy it! This is a lovely side effect of my healthy journey!

My day isn't going to go as I planned it work- and errand-wise. But it has every sign of going as I've planned it food-wise! I was wise this morning and thought out what I would eat today. I have something to pack with me. And sugar isn't coming along for the ride. I don't like amusement park roller coasters. And I don't like sugar roller coasters. Sugar puts me on a mood roller coaster.

Speaking of coasters, coasting is "moving easily without using power." The gravity of this situation—coasting—is that it goes in a downward direction, but not on the scale. I like the sense of power I have when I'm not in the clutches of sugar. I like the feeling of control I have when it isn't in the driver's seat. (I could say something about standard and automatic here, but maybe I'll just park that thought for now.)

So while my day won't go as I planned it, I'm not going to coast through it. I'm moving forward with power. I'm moving with good foods that have been carefully selected and measured—considering the sugar potential of each. It's all about being in control.

Some days I wrote multiple entries, and this was one of them. I don't remember if the titles were meant to go together, but I can see a connection!

PUSHING IT
April 18, 2013

My daughter-in-law is expecting my first grandchild! I've heard two due dates for her. One is today, and the other is Sunday. I've given birth to three children of my own, and none of them arrived on any of their due dates. But still. It's pretty exciting to think that today or tomorrow (or even next Wednesday or not) could be my grandson's birthday!

I'm writing a lot today, because that's what's working for me to stay away from sugar. I want to be sugar-sober for this wonderful experience and beyond. So, I'm keeping to my plan of writing my way through eating urges. It could be called crazy, but the point is it's working! I think it's a bit funny that I'm a writer (sort of), and my son's mother-in-law is a knitter. We're on pens and needles waiting for this baby to be born. Well, that's pushing it a bit. We're still waiting to hear that labor has started! Perhaps I should breathe!

Anyway, there's a little weight-loss related analogy with this. I know I've been impatient to get to my heart goal weight. In some ways I've been impatient. And in other ways I've acted like I never want to get there. The thing is that I took almost nine months to get to my healthy-weight range after I started the process. When I've just made the effort to work my tools of healthy living, the weight has come off as a side effect. And I've emerged as me—out of the layers of excess poundage I used to hide behind.

When I was in labor with my first child, I was wanting things to hurry along a bit. I was already a week past her due date and super sensitive to every twinge. I thought I was further along in the labor-and-delivery process, and I thought I could hurry things up by advancing to the next stage of breathing! That wasn't so smart. It made me more tired, and she wasn't ready to show her cute little face to us for another few hours.

Lesson to me: Don't try to rush things when you really don't have control over a situation—it's exhausting and frustrating and not necessary.

Okay. That's enough for now. The time will come when it comes. It's not pushing it to start fixing dinner now. And when the right time comes, I think I'm going to enjoy pushing a grandbaby carriage!

I've heard that knowledge is power, and I think the more knowledge I found about myself, the more power I had to be the real me.

TRYDAY?
April 19, 2013

Sometimes it's appropriate to try. And other times it's best to just do it. This past Tuesday was the day that I stopped trying to get out of the mess I was in with sugar. And the day I did my first day of sugar (re)detox. And the next day and the next day and the next day have been good. I haven't been trying. I've been doing.

My husband and I were talking about the mind games that happen with a quick loss. It's easy to think it's okay to eat just a little more and not pay attention to portion control and then graze through the evening. All of that. It's easy to think I could then just pop the extra weight off when the clothes start getting too tight. The problem I've proved too many times is that my yo-yoing has trended in an upward direction.

Trying to do better is what's gotten me there. Because trying seems to give my brain an out. (*Well, I tried to be good all day, but that just looks so good. I'll try again tomorrow.*) So I'm not trying anymore. I'm doing this. I've done it before. And I can, and I am doing this again. Today. And yesterday. And tomorrow. And if I run into an obstacle? It won't be because I'm just trying. I'll just do it—around or over or through. Even if I have to pick myself up again in the process. I'm doing it.

Do It Day. Or maybe Just Do It Day. In Greek mythology, Nike is the goddess of victory.

Sometimes a challenge makes all the difference.

CHALLENGE POINT
April 26, 2013

Early in my online experience, I found that I was spending a huge amount of time in the WW blogging community. I would read and write when I felt like eating. And usually it helped me get through the moments (there were a lot of them) and enabled me to wait until mealtime to eat. At a certain point, though, I realized I couldn't really live like that. I had things to do and places to go. Spending copious amounts of time at the computer wasn't helping with that. Right around that time, another blogger posted a challenge. It was to make up a mini challenge for a week and do it. It was a simple, nonbossy challenge. It was self-directed and exactly what I needed.

I challenged myself to get at least twenty minutes of exercise before blogging. Initially, I did the minimum. And possibly for the first time in my life, I rewarded myself for exercising with writing instead of eating. (I remember stopping at the grocery store for a treat after exercise class. I probably consumed twice as many calories as I'd burned, and I gained weight while I exercised three times a week.)

I continued the challenge, and most days, I met it before I wrote. I didn't check in to the challenge site much again. But that was okay, because it did what I needed it to do. And I'm still thankful to that fellow blogger for nudging me into exercising regularly.

Now, because I might burst if I don't include it: I am the proud grandma of a brand-new baby boy! I'm looking forward to meeting him tomorrow. I did my first exercise class as a grandma this morning.

One strategy to stay on my plan had to do with having appropriate snacks with me if I needed them while I was away from home. This thought ended up in a poem!

FOODS WiTH APPEAL
May 1, 2013

I think a big deal
Is to find the appeal
In fruits with a built-in wrapper.

They're easy to pack
For a pick-me-up snack
And assist with my quest to be dapper.

I have to be sure
(For my sugar-management cure)
To be certain to eat them with protein.

Bananas with string cheese
Apples with almonds, please.
That's how it works for Maureen!

Nancy Reagan built an antidrug campaign around the slogan, "Just say no!" I am old enough to remember that without consulting Google. It made a great seed thought for a post.

N.O.
May 10, 2013

There is something about the word *no*. Sometimes it's hard to say. And other times, it's way too easy. The second case usually involves a two-year-old. But I'm thinking about the first case for me and food.

Sugar: N.O. (Narcotics Opportunity. Just say, "NO!")

Chips: N.O.O. (Never Only One)

Family Gatherings: N.O. (Necessary Obligation? Nice One. Diffuse it with a compliment, so the excess calories won't complement your hips.)

Between Meal Eating: N.O. and N.O. (Not Overweight and Not Obese—partly because of saying NO to between-meal eating.)

Not Exercising: N.O. (Need Oxygen! or Nylons Overrated [control tops can only do so much])

This is only a partial list. I'm going to end it with a positive reminder to tell myself: Y.E.S. You're Eating Slim!

Although the slips could be considered discouraging, I found it encouraging that I kept writing and kept trying to find the light side, even if I was down about the mouth and up about the scale.

SEUSS-SAYING
May 16, 2013

I woke up this morning in a not-so-great mood.
I knew it was just about (all about) food.
I started to grump
Sort of turn to a frump
I knew it wouldn't be good.

It starts with a nod to
The Cat in the Hat
And goes on from there
With thoughts about fat.

Without further ado
For me and you too
(If you want, you can read it.
That's up to you.)

Look at me! Look at *me*!
Look at me *now*!
It is fun to be thin
But you have to know how.
(That's what I said
With a tilt of my head
And not with a bow.)

When all of a sudden
(But not really, I say)
Things started to crumble
And fall out of play.

Blueberry crumble
Or streusel-topped pie
Nothing's off limits
With a sugar-based high

Or low, for that matter
With a laugh and then cry
Why did I eat that?
Why did I? W*hy*?

Up on the scale
And the numbers are rising
The negative self-talk
The feel of despising.

But still the call
Of sugar is strong.
A nice piece of fruit
Or some bread can't be wrong.
(Or maybe it *is*—for me to be strong).

I have to stay balanced
On good healthy guidelines
Or, splat, I will find
Myself on the sidelines

(A place of regret—
Not cheering folks on—
A place of self-pity—
Maureen or moron?)

Now *stop*! I say, "*Stop!*"
All is not lost.
There is some recourse
But it comes at a cost.

I'll clean up my mess
With some help from my friends.
They can help just so much
But on me it depends.

What do I want?
Attention and fanfare?
Or genuine healthy
And knowing that I care.

I think it's the latter.
The former's a splatter:

Pride goes before a fall.
Rules get sloppy.
Resolve goes floppy.
What do *I* want?
It's my call.

I've proven to me
Once more(een), I see
I can't afford to be lax.
I know what to do
And, perhaps, so do you!
It's a matter of facing the Fats!
No head in the sand.
Denial's not grand.
Pick my face up.
Get back on the tracks.

When I track what I chew-chew
This train goes from moo-moo
Away from the grazing!
Action! Not lazing!
Perhaps it will lead to gazelle?
No.
A deeper thought
And here it is:
I simply will be well!

I don't think I could be classified as a true hunter-gatherer, but I know I used to hunt for chocolate and gather sweets. There's something fishy about that, I think.

BIG GAME TRACKING AND THE SCALES
May 20, 2013

I've been struggling with the official number I'm supposed to be at for monthly weigh-ins. I had gotten down to see the 150s on one unofficial weigh-in. I was two-tenths of a pound away from my seventy-five-pound star. And something happened. A little at a time. And to my horror, I've actually seen the 180s a couple of times in the last month. It's a good thing I checked and put the brakes on. Who knows where I'd be by now if I hadn't.

I think part of the problem was sugar and stress eating. But a bigger part of the problem was *comparing myself to the wrong thing.* I wasn't measuring up to how I felt. I was measuring against other people.

I don't look too bad. I'm smaller than her. I'm much smaller than I used to be. It's not about other people's size or how big I used to be. It's about how I feel in my skin and in my clothes right now. It's about how I feel in my head and my heart. I'm seeing that pretty clearly right now.

We talked about surprising food values at the WW meeting today. Reduced-fat blueberry muffins are pretty much a sham when it comes to the healthy choice options. That led me to think about big-game tracking. Like mousse. Or bear claws. Or elephant ears. Or even lobster tails à la Mike's Pastry in Boston. My conclusion is: It's better to know what you're tracking before you get to it, because it could turn on you and cause a lot of damage.

Almost everything I experienced sparked a weight-loss or sugar-management analogy. The honors breakfast at my daughter's high school didn't disappoint.

NOTICING THE GOOD
May 24, 2013

One of the things we heard at the high school honors breakfast this morning was that too often in our society, bad things are sensationalized and paid too much attention. The purpose of today's assembly was to celebrate and recognize the good that was going on every day in my daughter's high school. They gave credit to the families and friends of the students and also to the students themselves.

A good portion of each class receives honors or high honors. The principal said that it had been suggested that too many students received the honors because of grade inflation. But he disagreed with that thought. He cited the AP distinctions the school has received. The school is in a respected list of top schools in the country. I don't know what the criteria are for those awards, but I don't think it's anything to sneeze at. The honors don't say that these students are perfect or that the school is perfect, but they recognize that there is a lot of good going on that is worth noticing.

I started thinking about honor roll. And I got *on a roll* with WW stuff.

I'm noticing that I wanted to exercise today. And although I couldn't do it as much as I wanted to or in the manner that I prefer, I did it. And then I had an honorable breakfast. One that looked good, tasted good, and was worth sitting at the table for. I ate it in a way that I could appreciate the visual and taste senses of it. It was a collection of foods in the right combination for my body's best interest and performance. And that's probably enough to say about that.

I've spent a lot of time over the past months noticing failures and feeling not so great about them, but I've come to realize that I need to notice the good things more. There are quite a few of them, and they're worth noticing.

A wise friend of mine once said that it's important to keep balanced. Looking at the sky all the time could cause a person to trip in a pot hole of reality. Looking down all the time could cause a person to trip in despair. Well, my friend said it much clearer than that. But this is how I remember it. And will keep remembering it. For good!

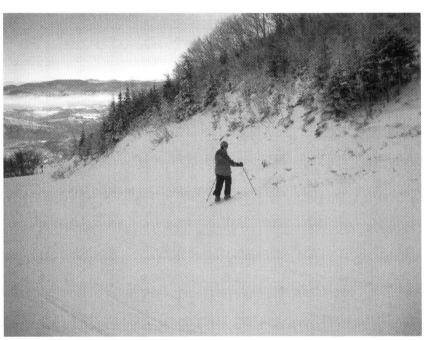

My original profile picture on the WW site featured an indistinguishable me in a men's extra-large ski jacket against the large bluish backdrop of a ski mountain. Basically, it's a point in blue. It's me hiding in my obesity.

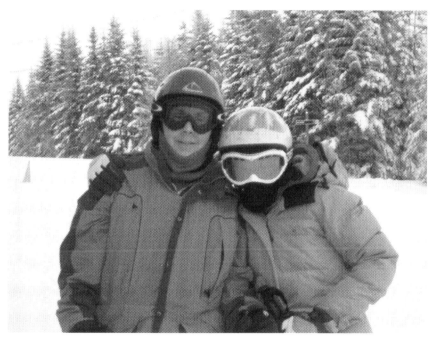

Ski trip in 2009.

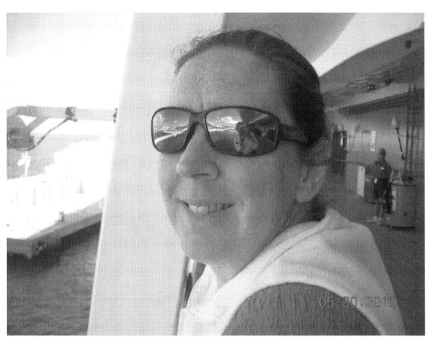

My husband and I took a cruise for our 25th anniversary in 2010. I lost some weight before we went. We used the stairs instead of elevators. I controlled my food intake until the last day. It was the beginning of another upswing on my size.

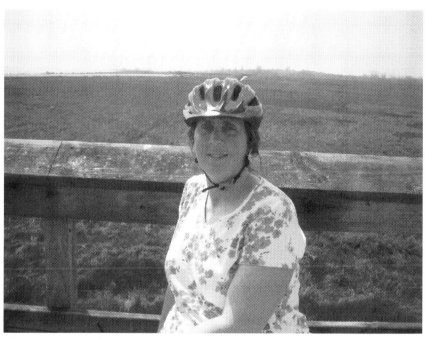

This picture is from a bike ride a year later. We were celebrating our 26th anniversary, and I remember I was trying to lose weight before my son's wedding.

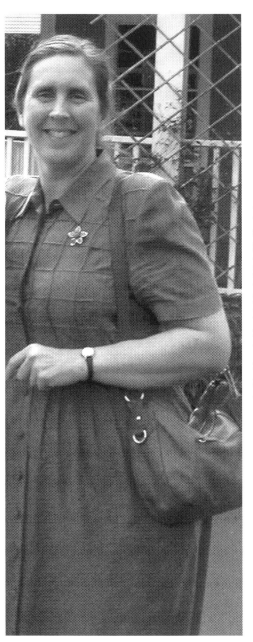

Here I am on June 17, 2011, as the mother of the groom. Smiling because it was a happy day. Smiling because I had convinced myself that it didn't matter what size I was because the day was not about me. I remember thinking that it just might be my lot to be obese. It seemed impossible for me to lose weight and keep it off.

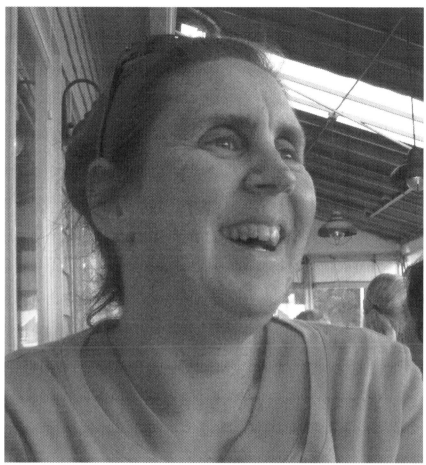

After the reception, we changed and went for a walk by the shore. My daughter caught this picture while we were waiting for supper. I remember huffing and puffing as we walked. But I had decided that if I couldn't get rid of my fat, I was not going to let it get in the way of my being happy.

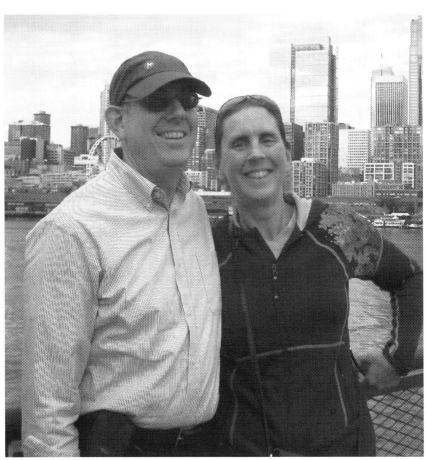

Fast forward to June 2012. I had been working at reducing my sugar for a little over seven months and working my WW tools for six months. I was still overweight, but I was in control. This picture is my husband and me on a ferry near Seattle.

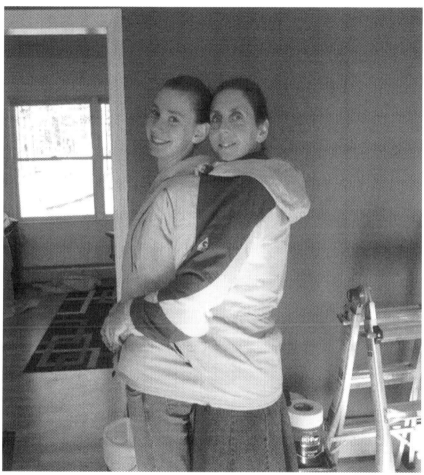

Later in 2012, I dragged out my old ski jacket from my heaviest weight and zipped my daughter and me in it.

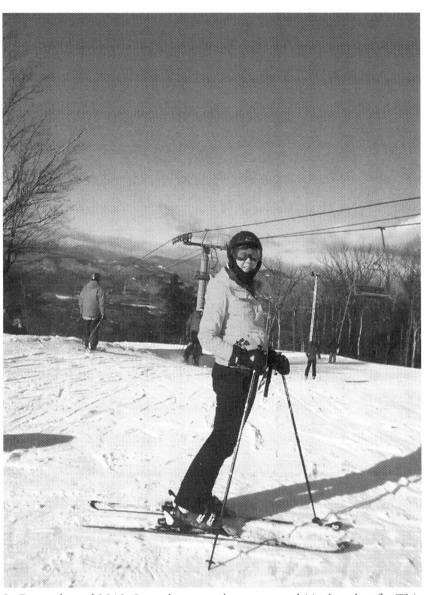

In December of 2012, I was happy to have a new ski jacket that fit. This time, I wasn't afraid to be recognized in the picture.

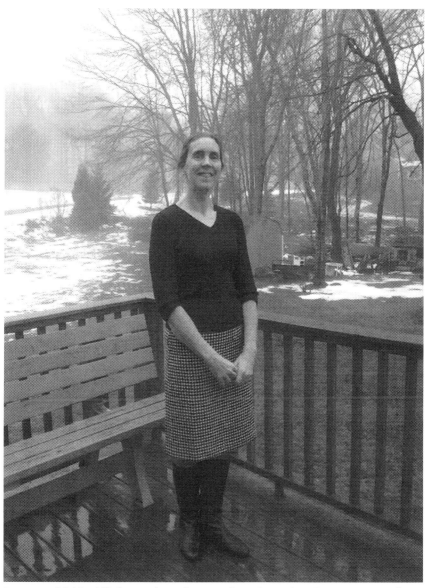

January 2013. All dressed up for my One Amazing Day event to share my weight-loss experience at the WW center. I didn't know it was the beginning of a struggle to really accept my sugar addiction as I tried to maintain my healthy weight.

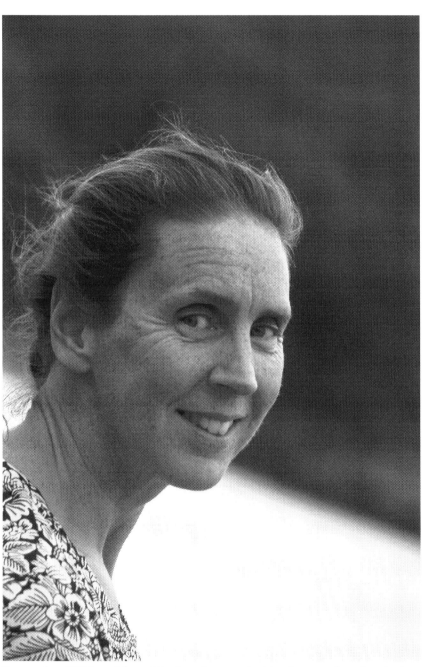

September 2015 and free. My daughter took this picture of me just before I submitted my manuscript for line editing.

PRACTICE MAKES PREPARED

Knowing I'm Not Perfect, but Finding Out I'm Ready for a Test

All of the previous posts were like practice for what happened next. My dad had a major stroke, and life as I thought I knew it changed drastically. Blogging became even more of a safety net in my quest to manage my sugar addiction and keep a clear mind.

UPDATE ON A DOWNDATE
May 26, 2013

My dad had a stroke yesterday (Saturday). He's had some hospitalizations over the last while, but not like this one. This has affected his speech and mobility. His sense of humor still shows through, and we're thankful for all the positives we can notice. But it's a serious problem. There are a lot of unknowns. And stress.

To back up a little, on Friday night, my husband and I took our youngest daughter to stay with my folks for the weekend. We were planning to return on Sunday evening to stay overnight and be with my folks for a Memorial Day get-together at their home. When we arrived Friday night, my dad greeted me with a big smile and said, "I just finished catching up on your blog!" (He loved to read what I wrote along with the comments other people wrote in response. We had conversations about the people we only knew by username and written personality. I think he was one of the first people to suggest I turn my blog into a book.)

Anyway, we had a lovely quick supper with my mom and dad, both of our daughters, and the two ministers who were staying with them. My dad was telling stories and making us laugh. My husband and I returned home for our anniversary weekend. Early Saturday morning we got the call that my dad was in the emergency room. We headed back to see him and my mom. It was a shock to see the effects of a major stroke on this strong man who had just the day before been weed whacking in the pouring rain to get ready for the get-together. Life and death looked pretty close, and there was no way to know how close.

Last night I gave my mother a ride to the hospital. My younger daughter accompanied us. And when my daughter wondered if she really should have gone (none of the others of her generation were there—just me and my siblings), I told her it was really good that she came with me. Her just being with me prevented me from stopping at a store on the way home to get a sugar hit.

I know I have a problem with eating in secret. It helps me understand that this is an addiction that I'm dealing with. My daughter's presence helped me know that drowning in sugar would not solve any problem. It might make me think I felt better while I was eating it or drowning in it as an escape from reality, but it wouldn't make anything better. The reality would still be that my dad was very sick and possibly wouldn't live very much longer.

When I posted about my dad's stroke, I had a huge outpouring of care and prayer from my online WW friends. They really cared, and I appreciated all of their supportive comments. I think the value of writing about my feelings increased dramatically through this experience.

HOME AGAIN
May 27, 2013

I've had some unplanned trips that I didn't trip on. And this weekend I had a few more. This time the catalyst was my dad's stroke. I've appreciated all of the thoughts and kind comments on my wall and posts. And I'm thankful for all the help I've felt from far and near.

My dad is showing some improvement. He can write on a whiteboard when his voice just can't convey his thoughts (which are very clear). His sense of humor is helping us cope.

The get-together that had been planned at my folks for today was canceled, but my son and his family met us there for a modified cookout that included a Greek yogurt dill dip, potato chips, fresh pineapple, carrot sticks, and hot dogs. My mom keeps cookie-dough balls in the freezer, and my two daughters baked some of them for dessert.

I had packed a sandwich that I ate at the hospital, and after holding my grandson while everyone else had lunch, I decided to have a hot dog with part of a bun. And a few chips. It could have been counted as the third meal of the day, but it was closer to lunchtime than supper. On our way home, we stopped at Wendy's where I got a plain baked potato that I ate with lots of pepper and one packet of salt. It was a bit underdone, but that worked to slow the pace of eating it.

As I entered in my food for the day, I was happy to see I had eaten a reasonable amount. I had no need to eat more, and no wishes I'd eaten less! Weigh-in is tomorrow. I'll see if the hot dog did damage or not. No matter. I'll keep going.

My dad was moved to a rehab hospital after a few days in a regular hospital. I continued to find things to blog about in my quest to work my tools.

REHAB HOSPITAL
June 3, 2013

If you pick out some letters and rearrange them a bit, there's HOPE in my title. And sometimes I have to look a little closer in certain situations to see the hope. But it's there.

I'm happy to feel like there's hope for my dad's recovery from his stroke. Some of the hope is recognizing what has to be regained and worked on. And some of it is doing therapy to reconnect the pathways that were disconnected. He has very clear thinking, and his sense of humor is sharp. I asked him about a rug kicker today, and he proceeded to draw a makeshift one to craft from a board. His thought process for that is a lot clearer than mine.

Right now, I'm thinking about my recovery or rehab from sugar addiction or sensitivity. Whatever it's called, there are many similarities to alcoholism in the condition. For some reason, my brain and body chemistry have a tendency toward that, and the only way for me to deal with it is to rehabilitate myself. I didn't have to go to a hospital, but I did find hope in the book *Potatoes Not Prozac* and the WW eTools.

I joined WW to use the tracker and blogging tools. It's worth repeating. A few times. Maybe quite a few times! In using the tools, I got rid of a lot of excess weight. I was logging my foods and blogging my moods. Eventually, I started jogging my moves!

I made it back to lifetime status in October 2012. But then I seemed to get to a slippery slope of maintenance. I was slipping up with my original plan of logging and blogging my way with the sugar guidelines I had learned. Reaching a certain weight didn't take away my sugar addiction. I've proven that I still need the guidelines to keep feeling healthy in my mind and my body.

I'm choosing to be thankful that I have learned these things. In following the guidelines and using the tools, I've had hope fulfilled. That kind of sounds like GOAL. But only in the sense that it stands for Going On And Living. Continuing to use my tools.

I typically wrote my blog posts in silence or to the swish of my washing machine, which was next to my computer. But it occurred to me that I needed to listen. Even in the silence.

LISTENING POINTS
June 4, 2013

A few months ago, I was listening to an audiobook in the car. It was Dale Carnegie's *How to Win Friends and Influence People*. It's not a new book, but it has some great information in it that's worth listening to. Actually, one of the key things I learned was that listening is huge in establishing relationships.

Listening has been a big deal in working with my dad post-stroke. Well, it has always been a big deal with my dad. He is a great storyteller. (He is a great listener too.) Right now, his speech is affected. His thought process isn't. He knows what he wants to say, but it's hard to get the words out so that they can be understood. But it's important for us to listen and make the effort to find out what he is saying. Because it's a big part of how we can help him feel better.

Last night, I stayed with my dad in the rehab hospital. It was an interesting experience, and partway through the night I realized that although one of the caregivers was really nice and wanted to be helpful, he didn't always listen. He seemed more interested in talking. And as I listened to him, I felt a little frustrated that he wasn't taking the time to really listen to my dad. Instead, he was assuming things. I think we finally got to the same page, but it was a lesson to me about listening. And I can be a better listener because of it.

Because I'm fairly tuned in with my use of this blog tool, I'm thinking that a big part of my weight-loss/good-health journey is listening to or taking in information and processing it. Listening is writing my foods down in the tracker and paying attention to what my body is trying to tell me when I eat certain things. It's paying attention to the scale when it shows a trend in the right or wrong direction. It's not the scale's fault that it's telling me a certain number. It is just reporting what my body is telling me if I would only listen to it.

For years, my body tried to tell me sugar was my enemy. And perhaps it was a stroke of luck that I ran across the *Potatoes Not Prozac* book that helped me listen to understand what I needed to do. And as I did just that, I listened to my body thank me for taking care of it. The voice of sugar became less alluring, because I realized it didn't care one iota about me. It was just good at talking and assuming I would just keep reacting to it in the same way I always had.

When I realized the dangers of sugar, it was easier to stick with listening to my body. Sugar assumes I'm going to cave to it. Sugar expects me to go along for the ride and need more and more for that fleeting feeling of comfort, which is actually a lie.

That segues into another thought I had during my night in the hospital. Sugar tells me a lie. When I get victory over that—insert the *V*—I know what it is to live and not diet!

That's all for now. They are thoughts I had in the middle of the night, and I listened.

I spent time at my folks doing yard work, and I also spent time at the rehab with my dad. I was back in the neighborhoods where I'd grown up. They were the neighborhoods I knew well in the days before I knew sugar was poison to me. I think locations can be a trigger, but they don't have to be pulled.

JUST FOR THE RECORD
June 6, 2013

I thought of a new spin on this earlier this morning. I had eaten a mini Larabar without knowing how much it would cost in my tracker. And then I ate two more. They are such cute little things, and they are rather tasty without having a lot of junk in them. The ingredients are all real food. But because my purpose in joining WW online was, and is, to use the tools, I entered the nutritional values to find the tracking value. It ended up being a lot, but it went in the record because it went in me.

When I don't record my food—when the record is broken—what's playing out gets stuck in a repeat. It might be a yo-yo pattern or a general plateau that begins an upward spiral. However it gets broken, it impedes forward movement in my continuing success story.

Back to the Larabars. They were in the clearance bin at the grocery store near my parents' home. They were marked down to five cents apiece, and I bought almost all of them—more than fifty. I saw them as a good thing to put in lunch boxes. I thought it might be nice to have a stash for my mother at the rehab hospital. They're enough to take the edge off real hunger. There are times when that's important but there's nothing decent to eat. My mother knows herself, and she knows how to eat appropriately for good health. I didn't think the Larabars would pose a problem for her.

For me, I have to be careful to not break the record. Keep recording. Keep being aware. I can't afford to slide into a "scratch that" mode (as in: I ate it, but I'm going to pretend I didn't), because my body is keeping the record with amazing precision and will respond accordingly. The bars may have been cheap for my wallet, but the price my body pays for eating them is constant no matter how expensive or inexpensive they might have been.

Keeping the record helps me not be surprised with my results. Keeping the record helps me balance how I spin my exercise and maybe record some more.

After I wrote about the Larabar, a blogger friend made a comment that inspired this post. She said, "Knowing you as I do, I think you could rise to the challenge of the Larabar and create the 'Maur Bar' for lesser you." After a few minutes that actually included considering eating another of the mini Larabars, I had a response for her wall.

THE MAUR BAR
June 6, 2013

The Maur Bar!
It's done!
An empty wrapper
For the best bar: None!

An empty wrapper would provide the satisfaction of a purchase and the satisfaction of not consuming empty calories or even nutrition-packed but not needed calories. This empty wrapper could represent a non-scale victory! There could be an encouraging message on the inside of the wrapper.

I can almost see it for sale now: a slightly puffy wrapper made of almost-impossible-to-open Mylar. It wouldn't be thrown away once opened, but stashed in a purse to accumulate as visual reinforcement of how well a person is doing resisting temptation to eat. I almost wonder if I should be writing about it, because it's such a brilliant idea!

I'll have you know that I didn't eat another mini Larabar just now. But that's just on my say so. If I'd had a Maur Bar, I could have had the empty open wrapper to show my success in not eating anything!

This new thought raised the bar, and I was on a roll!

MORE ABOUT THE MAUR BAR
June 7, 2013

My venture into weight-loss aids
Has given me lots of thought
For the value of a little help
With victory in battles I've fought.

The urge to buy a little treat
Just a taste sensation really
A reward of sorts in the middle of the day
But too costly to eat them freely.

I came up with an alternate bar
With a challenge to my head
An empty wrapper only
A non-scale victory instead.

A simple visual reminder
Of what just might have been
If the wrapper had been really full
And the points to count were ten.

The Maur Bar to the rescue!
Maur wrappers in your tote

Might mean vict'ry on the scale
Instead of a sugary bloat.

I've had a bit of fun with this
But there might be a serious side
And reason to spend some cold, hard cash
For a wrapper with nothing inside.

What is the true cost of empty snacks?
In the course of a weight-loss journey?
Working so hard for the lose and all
But it seems like a yo-yo tourney.

I could be called delusional
But perhaps there's a market for this
A tool that might help a struggler hold on—
To work toward goal and not miss.

The goal I mean is the new, improved version:
Going On And Living!
Continuing to use the same proven tools.
They work every day with thanksgiving!

So what do you think?
Would anyone bite
For a bar like this
Or the Maur Delight?

The second version
Not filled with plain air
But with helium
Like a balloon at a fair!

The Mylar wrapper's
Quite hard to get loose.
Resistance training
For double-hand use.

It's like playing
A personal tug-of-war
To tear open the wrapper
To get at no bar.

But the prize!
Yes, the prize!
When you open your eyes:
You've not eaten a thing that will pad up your thighs!

And there's proof!
It's no spoof!
(Well, perhaps, partly a goof.)
An on-program day has not just gone *poof*!

I'm just about sold on this!
Order a case!
It will help bridge the gap
To that thin healthy place!

My blog topics might be compared to a roller-coaster ride. Perhaps that could suggest I had wild mood swings, but I really believe that exploring and explaining my thoughts and feelings prevented the type of swings I'd had under the influence of sugar. In reading over what I wrote, the general feeling is positive. In my analysis, that's a good thing.

GETTING AWAY WITH IT
June 13, 2013

There's a thought process that goes along with my title as if there is a way to avoid consequences of an action. And then there's the idea of closet eating, as in getting away with IT. Getting away from all other eyes (possibly with a blindfold or at least with one's head in the sand) and eating something. Ingesting Temptation. The problem with me eating things in secret is that they are proclaimed on my hiptops and tend to affect my mood in a negative way.

Eating in secret, or just contemplating it, is a red flag to me that I'm in addict mode. I need to review my tracker to see where the sugar or processed foods or just too many carbs with not enough protein have crept in. And if I haven't been tracking, it's a sign to me to press the detox button. Now. Do not pass go. Do not collect one last sugar hit. It's not a go-to-jail situation. It's get out of jail and stay out. Because, for me, living under the influence of sugar is like a prison.

The way I'm trying to see it is: Getting (as in understanding) away with it. As in: Be gone! Don't have it around. If something is proving to be too much temptation (as in irresistible), it's less expensive to throw it away and be done with it than to risk eating it and having to pay consequences. It needs to be a proper disposal (not a human garbage disposal). I think I get it.

This post has another shout out to the online WW community of support.

INSPIRED AND INCITED INSTEAD OF EXPIRED AND EXITED
June 19, 2013

I've found that my uncontrolled addiction to sugar tends to want to give up, give in, and get out. So I'm thankful that I've learned to recognize some of the warning signs that I'm on dangerous ground. One of them is a reluctance to log (my food), jog (my moves), and blog (my moods). It's not always in a certain order, but they seem to trigger each other.

That voice of despair
That's shaped like a pear
And leads to moods bottoming out—
Needs to be hushed
And the attitude flushed
Before it's a full-fledged pout.

All that it takes is a kind little word
(Or sometimes a kick in the pants).
The music restarts, I get in my place
And I find that I'm back in the dance!

Yes, sugar coats the picture
With a bunch of stuff that's false.
But all it takes is three small steps
And it's possible to waltz!

Logging, jogging, and blogging.
That's what works for me.
Using the WW online tools
With *Potatoes Not Prozac* by K. DesMaisons, PhD.

It helps me keep my G.O.A.L. in sight!
To make food choices that are right!
Community support—we are so tight!
To abandon this would be a sad fright.

I love the access: morning, noon, and night.
To write my thoughts instead of bite.
And read other thoughts united in this fight.
Suggesting what to do in the most perplexing plight.
Or lists of NSVs that bring me great delight.
Repeating what works because it's never trite.
Knowing that just doing it will work and not just might.
Seeing the present and future are bright.
(As long as I stay away from my Kryptonite!)

The Kryptonite reference was given to me by a fellow blogger. She knew, sometimes better than I did, that sugar took away my powers to work my tools for being healthy. The next post picks up on another part of Superman!

ESCAPE
June 20, 2013

I suppose that escape could be something Superman wears. My real title should probably be landscape, but I was able to go on a little journey in my brain with this title.

Yesterday I did some weed whacking at my parents' home. Today I mowed the lawn and did some weeding by hand. Just as I was reaching for one of the little green interlopers, I froze and then drew my hand back. It was baby poison ivy! By not touching it, I have escaped certain misery.

I did the rest of the nonpoisonous weeding and then called my mom at the rehab and asked about killing the poison ivy. Fortunately, my dad was able to tell her where I could look for the materials to get rid of it. What I've used in my yard comes premixed. My dad had concentrate and a spray thing to mix it in. Fortunately, I was able to figure it out and get to work.

I went on a rampage in the yard.
No poison ivy was safe.
I spotted the clusters and drenched them
With a careful, well-aimed strafe.

The thing about poison ivy is that it looks attractive and healthy if you're not aware of the damage it can do. And that led me to the thought for this post. When I was on the way home this afternoon, I decided to stop at a grocery store for a planned snack. I bought a half a pound of cooked shrimp from the fish market. And I bought some blueberries, bananas, and a store-made fresh fruit cup. I ate it all. I knew I needed volume. I chose healthy foods that I thought I could handle. And so far, so good. With all that fruit, it could possibly be a sugar fail. But I think I had enough protein and seltzer and control over the time I took to eat it to escape without damage.

I could have gotten a protein bar. Or some other packaged snack. Some of them look quite attractive. And healthy. But the amount of sugar in them is too dangerous for me to handle. And so I'm staying away from them. That's as drastic as I'll be with the sugar. And now I must go to bed and get some sleep. That's part of my escape plan. Exhaustion can be a trigger for sugar problems, and I just don't want that.

I continued to grapple with the ups and downs of trying to maintain a healthy weight. Instead of getting frustrated to the point of giving up and giving in to sugar, I continued to write and write and write. Maybe I thought one of those writes would eventually get it right? Or maybe I was just starting to understand that this was something I'd need to work with for the rest of my life.

YO-YO NO MO!
June 22, 2013

I feel like I've been flirting with a yo-yo problem ever since I reactivated my lifetime status back in October. I've managed to weigh in each month within my healthy range to keep getting free online tools. But I have been bouncing on the scale a bit. Sometimes alarmingly so.

When I weighed in for June, the receptionist made a comment about me not needing to weigh in again for eight weeks. And although that was a true statement, it wasn't a good statement for me to hear. Because I used it to trigger some poor choices—as if they were sanctioned by the fact that I didn't have to weigh in until the end of July. It's the truth.

The problem with me running with that comment was that it would cut out my use of a very important tool in my G.O.A.L. (going on and living) at my healthy weight. Like running with scissors, it had the potential for extreme danger. I'm not able to get to my WW meeting extremely regularly, but I've been careful to weigh in at home every Tuesday. And by the next Tuesday (my meeting weigh-in was Friday), I was up. Weigh way up. I said to myself it was okay. But it wasn't. I didn't blog much. I wasn't tracking food. I had excuses for why, but I simply wasn't exercising good judgment (or my body much either).

Some inability to focus and deal with some tough emotional situations reined me back in. Calm is better. Planned is better.

I have to keep using the tools. They're lifetime tools that I have been using since January 2012. Tools that I used to shed a lot of pounds and continue to use to keep them off. Logging, jogging, and blogging. It works. It pays! And I'm free!

In defense of another look at justification, it's a big deal to a sugar addict. There's a wedge-like quality to the word that resembles pie or cake or something fake. When I find myself wanting to justify, I have to ask why.

JUSTIFICATION. YET ANOTHER LOOK. JUSTIFIED OR JUSTAFRIED. OR MAYBE JUSTAFRAID.
June 24, 2013

This morning I was thinking about the word *justify*. And what stuck in my head is that it's extremely important for me to stop and think about *why* I feel like I need to justify something. Is it to try to beat the system? Or to make someone else feel better? Is it to make me feel better? And for that matter, *can* it do what I think it can do to deserve the thought of being justified?

There are things that can be justified. And then there are other things that are better justafried. I'm not talking about batter deep fried! When computers are fried, it means they're unusable and probably need to be thrown out. There are things that I'm better off just not using. I should consider them justafried to me!

Then there are things I'm just afraid to try. Perhaps it's for a good reason. I have learned a lot about myself over the past year and a half. There are some things that I am justified to be justafraid of. Like how sensitive I am to sugar. I'm sensitive to bee stings too. Even if I have an EpiPen on me, I don't play with stinging insects! And if I happen to get stung anyway, history has justified me being justafraid. Of course, I've survived all of the stings I've gotten. But because the next one could be worse, I don't have justification to not exercise caution!

I know that I have tools to get me back on track if I get into sugar for some reason, justified or not. I have survived several instances of this since I reactivated my lifetime status with WW last fall. But it's not something I can take for granted, so I exercise caution. Me using the WW tools is justified—right and reasonable.

I wasn't chicken to write about poultry subjects.

FREE RANGE VS. FREE REIN
June 25, 2013

I can't say I know much about free-range chickens and all that. Free range, in my mind, is the coinage at the bottom of my handbag. It still has boundaries, but it has more room than in my coin purse. I'm guessing that free-range chickens aren't cooped up and unable to move about, but have extra room to forage or whatever it is they do. It's not like they can just go and cross the road any time they want. But they have some range before they end up on the range.

Free rein seems more to me like without any control. Able to go full speed in any direction with no boundaries. Without control, in my mind, is what happens when I'm on sugar. My impulse controls weaken, and nothing is off limits. And it's ultimately a scary place, because I tend to not care in the moment. (Mom meant to do better, but ... oh well, there's always tomorrow. And then, lying in bed, later that night, I hit the addict's valley of shame and regret only to forget about it after the first sugar hit of the next morning.)

I could have been there today. I'm at my parents' house right now. Last night, after getting back from the rehab center, I went to the basement fridge and found the remains of a store-bought sheet cake. They were leftovers that were brought to my parents' home by someone else from some event. It wasn't something my mother would normally have around, but it was there. I actually touched the plastic cover, and then I recoiled as if it were a rattlesnake. I safely retreated back upstairs.

I've thought about that cake and all the frosting on it a few times since. But I've also thought about the aftereffects if I were to indulge. The sugar haze. The foggy thinking. The lethargy. The regret. The too-tight clothes. And the cycle I just got off again and don't want to get back on. It is easier than riding a bike—that sugar cycle. But there are no health benefits. There's a certain high and then a crash. With a call for more and more. That used to be me. More and more sugar. Highs and crashes.

But ultimately a downward spiral in health and mood. And an upward spiral on the scale.

I was tempted this morning to drag my finger through the frosting and pop some in my mouth, but again, the aftereffects flashed through my mind. That's what I focused on to give me the fortitude to just say no (or maybe whoa)! Free rein would have had me eating through a good deal of that cake by now. Free range has me writing a blog post about it. I'm working within the boundaries of my healthy eating. I'm not in the cooped-up quarters of a diet.

My mom and I talked about the leftover cake this morning. We both agreed that it would be a good idea to get rid of it. It has served the purpose for which it was bought. The fact that there are leftovers is just indication that there was plenty for any who wanted some at the event. That event is over, and so is any reason to keep the cake around. I'm going to get my hazmat gear on and take care of it.

Not all of my topics were from current events. Something triggered this college memory into a blog post that fit the moment.

MEMORiES
June 28, 2013

Way back in the eighties when I was in college, I remember walking by a dormitory. A stereo was blaring, and the beat was strong. I noticed I was walking to its rhythm. "*Boom. Boom. Boom. Boom.* Another one bites the dust. *Boom.*" I tried to alter my step but had great difficulty doing it. I recall feeling a little troubled—feeling controlled by the music. And that's where the memory ends.

The title of my post—as a song—evokes an entirely different mood. And that mood thing segues, or should I say swings, into my topic today. Or perhaps I should say topics, because my thoughts are swinging wildly too. This swing thing is sort of like the giant ones you see at a carnival or fair. But this one isn't fair. It's reality right now. There are a few things I'm having to deal with. One of which is a case of poison ivy that started breaking out on my face Wednesday. It is spreading, which is discouraging and upsetting. It's also very itchy. That is stressful, and it's not helping the tired thing I have going on.

There are good ways to handle stress and emotions and tiredness. I've done them for months at a time with good results. And in worse stress.

But yesterday I didn't. Maybe the poison-ivy outbreak was the last straw? Or maybe not. Yesterday I felt like I was trapped in the beat of an obnoxious song. *Boom. Boom. Boom. Boom.* Another big bite, I must. *Boom.*

I did so well with the hazmat suit and the leftover cake earlier in the week. I was feeling in control. But I didn't think I was too proud about it. As in, pride goes before a fall. As in, flat on my face. To bite the D.U.S.T. Discouraged, Upset, Stressed, and Tired. Or Dreaded Uncontrolled Sugar Temptations.

I didn't handle things very well yesterday. All my troubles weren't so far away. I'll just say that I ate as if I wanted to weigh five hundred pounds. I was wallowing and biting dust. I found enough resolve last night to go to the store for the right foods for today. My husband was wanting to do a three-day detox plan as a final push in his work's fitness contest. And fortunately, I was able to tap into his enthusiasm as a lifeline out of my dust. I got enough food supplies for me too.

This morning I went to Jazzercise class. The first routine was done in a circle instead of the regular format with the instructor facing us. That was almost enough to derail me. I like not having to think too much when I'm exercising, but this required a lot of brain exercise because instead of following the instructor's lead, mirror style, I was having to do the same as her. Some of my classmates were also mixed up. And instead of the usual order, there was chaos. I felt grumpy and annoyed.

Maybe the change up was what I needed. I toyed with the idea of quitting class early, but I didn't. And by the time the ending song came around, I realized I was no longer aggravated. I wasn't feeling defeated. Sure, I had some muscle fatigue, but it felt good. I was tired but energized. I'm actually feeling like I could go for a run today as another stress reliever. I feel like I've kicked the beat of "Another One Bites the Dust."

I'm not even going to try to justify another take on this thought. Here it is!

JUSTAVACAUTION
July 2, 2013

I'm heading into a vacation experience this week, and I'm just off of the rush of a sugar roller coaster. Vacation before the vacation? Seems like that could be a setup for a devastating event. Or maybe it's *de vast eating* event.

This morning I weighed in and recorded a ten-pound drop from last week. I could argue that it's not a real number. I'm not sure exactly what time of day I finally weighed in last week, but it was on Thursday instead of Tuesday, and I know that I was bloated from high-volume eating and poor food choices.

I was able to come to a screeching halt and turn the bus (that I was becoming) around with a three-day detox plan and increased exercise. I was in such a bad place on Thursday, though, that I actually bought and ate a Table Talk chocolate éclair pie while I was doing the grocery run for the foods to do the detox. My weigh-in was probably that evening, and it was my highest since getting back to my healthy range last August.

This morning, I used my tools and took a stroll back in my tracker. I found a wave pattern over the months since August. Interesting. It kind of goes with my yo-yo history. But to my credit, I've been able to weigh in, and I *have* weighed in every month since I reactivated my lifetime status last year. But the trend in the waves is higher. And I'm not interested in getting them to tsunami status, because that's devastating. De vast eating.

The think that I need to work on. (I started out with think, corrected the seeming typo to thing, and then realized think was the best word for here.) So, the think that I need to work on is maintain. A little ripple up or down is more in keeping with a lifetime goal. I've kept my tracker in weight-loss mode, because I really wanted to have my goal weight fifteen pounds lower than it is.

Obviously, that hasn't worked out the way I thought it would, so I need to think about this differently. The number is for the tracker. What I need to go on is how I feel and how I look. I have some clothes that don't fit as well as they did when I got them last fall. The reason I bought them is because I seriously felt like I would be wearing them for several seasons. Not winter, spring, summer, and fall. But for several winters, springs, summers, or autumns. (I just decided I like autumn better than fall, because this wave thing is too much like fall. Or fail.) So my goal is to wear those things comfortably and not play with numbers on the scale and in my tracker to think I'm doing okay.

I am feeling thankful for that tracker tool. Looking back at it shows me what I've really done, and in knowing that, I can deal with it. I can exercise caution. So I won't have a devasteating vacation!

We're going to the coast of Maine. And the main event will be my grandson! Not food. Sure, I'll enjoy fresh fish and maybe even some lobster with real butter. We'll have a partial kitchen and a full refrigerator stocked with healthy food. I'm not planning to coast on the waves and land on the rocks. And I'm not planning to swim with the sugar sharks. It's too painful. Even if there is an adrenalin rush in the process, it's just not worth it.

I'm not sure if I'll be online much. But I'll take the thought of *U* with me on vacation. Vaca*u*tion. Justavaca*u*tion. Not timid, but aware and informed. Staying healthy. Wearing my bathing suit. Not worried about how I look in it because I'm eating and living at lifetime!

It has been said that breakfast is the most important meal of the day. I think it's true.

BREAKFAST
July 3, 2013

Today was a busy day. I had to make two trips to the Department of Motor Vehicles, but I did okay. Partly because I had breakfast. It wasn't a typical breakfast, but it worked for me.

I started with shredded carrots and sliced onions sautéed in two teaspoons olive oil. I added one cup leftover broccoli, two Light Laughing Cow Swiss wedges, and a half a cup of egg whites. After I put the egg whites and cheese in the omelet pan, I turned the burner down low and took care of some e-mail business. The eggs were pretty much set when I folded them over. And the carrots had made a crispy crust. It was delicious. The cherries I had along with it were wonderful too.

Back to the DMV. I thought I had everything I needed, but after waiting in line for a long time to get a number (think deli counter), I found out I needed a copy of my husband's driver's license. Fortunately, I was able get that from my husband and get back to the DMV with about twenty minutes to spare in the two-hour waiting time for my number to be called. When I finally got down to the business of the day, everything was in order for my transaction to work.

I'm not sure what the lesson is here. Except maybe to eat breakfast, have patience, and don't give up.

Writing my feelings was the purpose for blogging. I'm not surprised that I eventually used the word as a topic.

FEELiNGS
July 5, 2013

In some parts of this fabulous country (Happy belated birthday, USA!), that word is pronounced *fillings*. In the flabulous state that I was in prior to this healthy-weight journey, feelings and fillings were very closely related. I'm talking about emotional eating. It doesn't help anything. It can provide some happy sensations in the brain for a fleeting period of time, but the consequences typically lead to poorer quality of life.

I've been thinking about feelings. I've noticed they can get in the way of good communication. Productive communication. They can get in the way of positive changes. And that can lead to problems. I was talking with someone the other day, and she made a comment, "That's a true statement. How does it apply to what you are trying to accomplish?" A light went on in my head. There was a potential for my feelings to get in the way of the objective, but because the focus remained on the objective, great things could happen.

I remember our drive to Maine and settling into a resort condo with our son's family and our younger daughter. By Sunday morning, the stress of prevacation had faded, and I had a better outlook in front of me.

NSV (NiCE SCENiC ViEW)
Monday, July 8, 2013

Sitting on the condo deck
With seagulls grooming the greens
Looking through yonder trees
What is that light that gleams?

The brilliant splash above the waves
At first a fuchsia pink
And as it rises higher—
A decided red, I think.

Sweeping strokes of color
Across the coastal sky

Shining a path on the water
On this lovely morn in July.

(Reflections from a Sunday Morning in Maine.)

A few days later, we got a call that cut our vacation plans short. We left the waves of the Atlantic Coast for the waves on my dad's heart monitor in the hospital. Both scenes a very real part of my life. I think writing was part of what kept me afloat. It was a life raft if I fell overboard or when my plans seemed to be sinking.

PLANS CHANGE
July 11, 2013

Which is why it is good to be flexible. I'm back from vacation early. I will be busy between home and helping my parents. I think of my online blogger friends often, and vacation was even better with *U* in it! Vacaution!

Because I was blogging, it was appropriate for me to tell my story over and over. It helped me remember why and how and where and what I was doing. But for a book, the repetition caused a glaze to the eyes, and glaze sounded too much like a sugar concoction, so I chopped a lot based on that. I think this entry was worth keeping, though.

E.A.T.
July 13, 2013

Emotional Awareness Tracking. I joined WW online to use the tracking tools. I wanted to eat enough to lose weight. And I wanted to track my feelings. Blogging has been a huge help that way. I have blogged my way instead of eating my way through feelings most of the time. And I will again. It is the right way to go for the right weigh at the scale and, more importantly, for the right way to feel.

There is much more to say about all of that. But not right now. For now, I am aware, and that has to be enough.

Battle scars don't stop the aging process.

MY FIRST WEEK AT FIFTY-ONE

July 22, 2013

For a while, I felt like fifty won. Something got into my brain and caused a sprain that just a few words couldn't really explain. Yes, I turned fifty-one and fell flat on my face. The very next day I was down in disgrace. Well, no, not disgrace. I still had my space. I still was aware. And still in the race. (Even though I felt like I was going backward.) I haven't had a lot of time to write a post in prose or rhyme. The thoughts come and go through my head. When I write, they come out half dead.

On Saturday I had a chance to walk up and down a hill that, in times past (as in, last year and more so the years before), would send me into huffing and puffing and wheezing. I didn't walk, though. I *ran*! It felt good. Even in my compromised condition of not-so-great eating over a few days.

Yesterday evening, my husband asked me if I wanted to go for a run. The temperature and humidity had broken a bit, and so we went. He kept asking how far I wanted to run. I kept not knowing. And by the time I did know, we had more than two miles to go to get back to the car. I probably walked a total of a mile and ran the rest for a total of six miles. I got an upper-body workout as well. The flies, even though I'd put bug spray on, were awful. I knew it was bad when I swept out my arms and felt seven distinct bugs hitting my palms. But we did it.

This morning, I got to my Jazzercise class and had a good workout. I still don't have a routine for this summer. And I may not be able to get one in place. There are many factors that change on a daily basis. But I can keep *aware*. And *beware* of an upward creep. Even if I can't always *see where* things are going to go that day.

I still don't have time to really write this post. But that's all right. I feel like I've righted myself on this trip around the sun. And the next fifty-one weeks at fifty-one are open for me to win!

Sometimes the word play is obvious, and other times it isn't. I think this next post was a little reminder to me to pay attention to what I was writing. I could write about all the right things, but if I didn't do them, well, I think that's where the hypocritical thought came in.

HiPPO CRITICAL
July 31, 2013

The timing is such
That I cannot write much.
But I thought of this phrase this morning.
When sugar's the crutch—
What I reach out to touch—
I think I should take a big warning.

I need
To take heed
To the things that I write.
To read and write blogs
Instead of a bite.

I think I'll revisit this idea in a few days. But for now, I'm going out to run.

A week later, I was ready to write again.

HiPPO CRITICAL REVISITED
August 6, 2013

I'm not being critical of hippos
They do what they're made to do.
But for me to not look like a hippo
I know I must track what I chew.

I've written a pile of blog posts
About simply using the tools.
But if I don't simply do that
I belong to a company of fools.

Fooling myself into thinking
It's okay for me just to know it.
And spout out wisdom that has worked for me
Then proceed to eat sugar and blow it.

Or perhaps I'll be careful with eating
And neglect my exercise.
Getting that out of balance
Is really not very wise.

It's the saying and doing and being
Balanced in body and soul
That work for the best along with the rest
And gives a safe sense of control.

The phrase of hippo critical
Is mainly just for a grin.
I'm thinking hypocritical
Works contrary to thin.

Now I have another thought
That's coming to my mind:
The concept of hypercritical
Is neither productive nor kind.

Expecting results
In too quick a time
Not giving credit
To reason (or rhyme).

Maturity and development
Come with their pace.
To rush one or the other
Makes me fall fat on my face.

Enough of the hippo critical.
Perhaps a better thought
Is thinking of Hippocratical—
Doing what one ought.

Although it's designed for doctors
Practicing medical art
It conveys a certain healthy respect
For doing what's right from the heart!

Although I'm not a doctor
In health care, or a nurse—
The Hippocratic text
Fits right in with this verse.

My healthiest conclusion
For my little blog
Practice what I preach
Don't be a hippo (or hog)!

I've been absent from this site for a few days. But I've not been absent from being aware of what I'm doing! I weighed in at my WW center on Wednesday last week. I had to pay, because I was just above my lifetime range. But I did it. I didn't just talk about doing it.

I am not able to use all of my usual tools because of circumstances beyond my control. Sometimes all I am able to do is be aware. I'm aware that I should be super careful the rest of the day. I'm aware that if I mess up, there is a new opportunity starting right now. I'm aware of how I'm feeling, aware that I'm human, aware that I need help, and aware of how to get it.

Believing I can. Be living. I can.

When I was packing for one of my trips to help my parents, I found some notes from when I couldn't get to a computer. Some nights I couldn't sleep until I had jotted down my thoughts. Once they were on paper, I could forget about them until I found the paper and decided to share.

MORE MUSINGS FROM MAUREEN
August 14, 2013

I need to trade in my forklift
For a one- or a two-pound weight
To transfer the bulge from my belly to arms:
And workout for what I just ate!

The benefits of a bicep curl
That doesn't end in my mouth
Offset the damage of fudge ripple swirl
When my intake control heads south.

The exercise thing is good, but it has to be moderated. I used to go to Jazzercise and then stop for a treat at the store on the way home. That wasn't good. I don't think it's a good practice to eat too much and then try to exercise it off, but sometimes it can stop a ballooning spiral of eating. I prefer to exercise *as* a treat most of the time now.

Another thing that can help me regain control is reading and commenting on blogs. I have to be careful to choose wisely, though. I like to read and write encouraging things like non-scale and scale victories. Sometimes the encouragement is just that the blogger showed up to write when it would have been easier (but in the long run more painful) to not. I have to be careful in my blogging to not get up from the computer and trip on the victory I just wrote about. It happens sometimes, but it hasn't been total defeat. I keep at it.

I just read a post from an online friend.
I've known her since last year.
She's struggling now with lifetime control
And I know very well that fear.

So in my comment to her thoughtful post,
I wrote a poem—a sort of toast?

The big deal I'm finding with maintenance
Is to keep my head out of the sand.
Staying aware
With a cautious beware
Will help things not get out of hand!

I too have struggles with lifetime.
But in that, there's a sign of life.
So I keep on trying a meal at a time—
To eat what's enough to suffice!

I noticed the political candidates posters for our town's election and put my own spin on the idea.

CANDIDATE FOR SUCCESS
September 4, 2013

To run or not to run. I'm electing to run. Last weekend, at the Labor (Day) Party, I looked like I was running away from everything I stood for (regarding healthy eating, that is). Except I did a lot of standing and sitting and not running.

I did a lot of eating too. And while I'm eating crow now, it was pig then. And all that goes along with a pig roast. It would have been good for me had I elected to cross the party line back into healthy eating as I was crossing state lines back home. But yesterday, I was still eating whole hog like a fat person even though I saw numbers on the scale that I hadn't seen for more than a year.

That was so yesterday, though. Today I'm a candidate for success. My meals are tracked, and I'm ready to go. On the road for a run.

Some of the posts I deleted were about running. Although they were a part of my journey, they were more of a by-product of me dealing with sugar addiction. It was a pretty big deal for me to sign up and train for a half marathon, and I found a way to relate it to my weight-loss, or whole-life, journey.

HALF MARATHON. FULL MAUREENATHON.
September 6, 2013

I'm feeling a little nervous this morning. The Hartford Half Marathon is coming up soon. Very soon. I'm a little off this week with my training schedule, but I'm still signed up for the race and I'll keep training. On race day, I'll do what I can and maybe a little more. Whatever happens with the half marathon, I'll be doing the full Maureenathon. I'm not racing, really. I'm aiming to be a finisher. I've read enough to know that there is no shame in walking part of it. I think that thought has to be part of my training.

My WW leader posted a really good comment on her Facebook page. I quote: "Time is going to pass no matter what you do. So what if it takes you two years to reach your weight loss goal? Three years? Four and so on. If every time things got tough and you quit—that is just extending those years on and on. STOP the madness and JUST KEEP GOING! Did you gain over the summer? SO WHAT—KEEP GOING!! Did you fall off the exercise bandwagon? SO WHAT—if your legs aren't broken right now you can move them, right? JUST STOP THE MADNESS AND KEEP GOING!!!!!!!!!!!!!!!! FOR ONCE, stop quitting!"

I've had my struggles with weight gain this summer. Actually, there is no struggle to gain weight. It goes on really easy. I struggle to get rid of it. And I get sick of the yo-yo game I play with myself. But the big victory is that I have not quit. And I will not quit. It's a lifetime thing.

I'm hoping it doesn't take me four years to finish the half marathon. But if it does, so what?! I'm going to keep on with my full Maureenathon. Logging, jogging, and blogging. But not quitting.

As I read and revised my blog posts to fit into this book, I thought about deleting things because they seemed too far out. But then I'd keep reading and recognize the value of the lesson I'd finally reached as I continued to play with my words. This post was one of the possible deletes. Perhaps the seat belt saved it.

CHANGING AROUND A FUNK (CREDITS TO SIMON AND GARFUNKEL)

September 11, 2013

Slow down, you eat too fast
You got to make the mealtime last
Just wolfing down the cobbler—groans
All too soon done and not feelin' groovy

Bad a, bad a, bad a, bad a … Not feelin' groovy

Hello blog post
What cha knowin'?
I've come to watch your AP's growin'
Got a reworked rhyme for you!
Doot-in' doo-doo
Feelin' groovy

I've got deeds to do
Promises to keep
I'm AP'd and WOW-sy and caught up on sleep
The morning is here and my day's up to me
Life, I love you
All is groovy

So really what I want to point out first is the groovy thing. I'm thinking about records and grooves. And eight-track tapes. Recording, or tracking, my food and exercise and moods is groovy. A good thing. And a good think.

I alluded to a crash in my status update yesterday. And this morning, I thought Catastrophic Reaction After Sugar High. I didn't feel like I had my seat belt on, but maybe I did. Because I'm here. I'm alive. Maybe a little bruised, but Self-Examination After Temptation Brings Excellent Lifetime Training. That works as a seat belt.

Speaking of seat belts, I had a great-uncle who didn't like the mandatory seat-belt law. He would pull the seat belt around and tuck it under his arm to avoid being stopped and ticketed by the police. No one was going to boss him around. He had the appearance of being restrained, but it was only an appearance. Had he been in a crash, it wouldn't have saved him.

When I only have the appearance of using my tools, I'm in a dangerous place. I have proved time and time again that I need to really use the tools in order for them to be effective. So perhaps, part of my seat belt is blogging. Truthful blogging.

My husband helped me see that last night. Part of my wake-up (and turnaround) was that what I was doing with sugar wasn't impacting only me. My frame of mind when I'm out of control with sugar has a negative impact on people I love. It's a big deal when a person realizes that irresponsible driving can destroy innocent lives. And it was a big deal for me last night to realize that my irresponsible eating was hurting more than me. I was in a dark enough place to not care so much about myself (sugar does that to me), but to possibly hurt someone else snapped the light on. I do care.

I also am old enough to remember cars without seat belts. And then they started becoming standard equipment. We had to learn to actually use them. My grandfather's car had seat belts, and he would exclaim, "Seat belts!" before starting the car. That helped us get to the point of automatic use. I didn't feel right if it wasn't properly in place. About the only way I wouldn't have my seat belt on is if I were distracted at just the right (or wrong) time. It doesn't take long for the uneasiness to set in and the problem gets resolved.

The point for me is that I think I allowed a distraction to get in the way last week. And then another. The warning signs came up. There was a halfway attempt to be restrained. But I wasn't completely honest, and I crashed.

I am amazed at how quickly my body packs on the pounds. But it's not that amazing, really. My body is always meticulously tracking everything I eat. It knows every step I do or don't take. It's watching me. And it is honest. And when I pay attention again, it has the potential to save my lifetime!

Whether I was exploring words or thoughts or just talking to myself, each blog post was a victory for me because I showed up to write it.

STRONG. END OF THE WEEK.
September 14, 2013

I couldn't decide if I should type week or weak. I'm feeling stronger than I was at the beginning of the week. But it's probably not the end of the weak for me. It will likely show up from time to time. But every time I get strong again, it's reinforcement that I don't have to stay weak! I think I might be able to string a week of strong days together. It's a goal for this week anyway!

There was a time to talk, and then there was a time I was sick of it. I blogged anyway.

TALK SICK. (OR TOXIC.)
September 19, 2013

I had a busy day today. I started with a great three-and-a-half-mile trail run with my seventy-year-old friend. (It was a beautiful, chilly fall morning.) Then I drove one hundred miles to see my parents. (My dad has made huge progress with his left side in the week and a half since I last saw him. He is also able to talk much more than he could.)

I cut the lawn and my dad's hair. (Using different tools.) I went on a mini shopping trip with my daughter. I weed whacked a section of yard that had been bothering my mother. (Take *that*, you weeds!) And I drove home. Another one hundred miles.

I could talk about losing a bunch of weight and maintaining the loss. Using the same tools. Except I'm not using all of those tools all that well right now. However, tomorrow is a new day. And instead of talking until I'm sick. I'm just going to do it. That is enough.

It helped me to look at words from unusual angles.

WHAT DO I DESERVE?
September 21, 2013

I was going to put *Entitlement* as a title, but then I thought people would wonder what my title meant. Deserve works better anyway.

Last week someone told me, "I don't deserve to be thin, and I don't deserve to be happy." Clearly, there was a problem, and I'm happy to say there have been positive steps away from this thought process. But the idea of deserve has been floating around in my head. And this morning while I was running, I was thinking about it some more.

What I'm thinking about is how to get rid of the extra weight I've found recently. Or maybe it's just how to be healthy again. I think it involves de-serving some things. It means not serving myself things that trigger a problem with my sugar sensitivity. It's not serving myself food in between meals unless it's a planned snack with protein and a start and stop time. And it's not serving myself food to try to take care of stress or emotional issues. In the process of de-serving it, I'll get what I'm working for!

The happy thing can involve some de-serving too. Sometimes I get in a twist about negative things. In weight-management speak, I suppose it could be a soft serve. But a good serving of reading positive blogs and making positive comments helps to de-serve the negativity. It's kind of related to the food thing, maybe food for thought. Feeding on negative thoughts leads me to a negative place. But looking for the positive and trying to feed on that leads me to a positive place. Like well-wishes, sometimes there has to be effort in digging the well, but it's usually worth it. Even if it's deep!

To change gears: My half marathon training is going well. The compression socks I got earlier this week helped immensely. I didn't get any blisters, and my toes didn't get messed up in my sneakers. I tried out a new hairstyle for running—a French braid crown. I liked how I didn't have to think about my hair flopping around or tugging on my scalp. I used a new sweat/headband and that was great too. No saltwater rivers into my eyes this time!

My total distance for running this week topped twenty-six miles. That's a full marathon. It took me from Monday to Saturday to do it. I'm feeling good. Everything I had to de-serve to get here was worth it!

RUNNING A HALF MARATHON

And Running Out of Free eTools

This next phase of my journey was about running out of my free lifetime passes and having to pay to use my online WW tools again. It was hard for me to think I'd lost that much ground and gained that much weight after having such a grip on what worked for me to be healthy in mind and body. I think this phase helped me realize I couldn't fix my sugar sensitivity. I just needed to accept it as my normal and work with it.

OVER WAIT
September 23, 2013

My numbers showed me as overweight
When I stepped up on the scale.
I had shrunk from facing hard, cold facts
But I wasn't the size of a whale.

Overweight wasn't nearly as bad
As if I had over waited
To return and use my collection of tools.
(Pride is way overrated).

If I'd waited as long as I did last time
I'd have rejoined the ranks of obese
But I went and I paid for a monthly pass
While wearing my size small fleece!

Although the season's officially fall
I walk with a spring in my step.
I'm working the tools with confidence.
I can do this! I will do this! Yep!

There's a popular phrase that says, "one day at a time." I was in the phase of one moment at a time.

MOMENTUM
September 24, 2013

It's moment by moment.
The um is a pause—
Is it really worth
A chomp with my jaws?

Actually, things are going well. I feel some momentum with doing the right thing. And the write thing. I have strung some successes together, and I'm wanting it to continue.

I did a three-and-three-quarter-mile trail run with my friend this morning. It was mostly single-track trail, but it had some rail-trail sections and then a section of paved road along with a gravel road. I think it could be called a trail mix. It was a good mix of up and down. And we shaved three minutes off our mile pace from last Thursday.

This momentum thing. I find it encouraging to have some forward movement. I'm taking charge. I can do this. I am doing this. There's something to finishing up a day having done what I could. It works better for me than: Mom Meant, Um. Meant to track it but forgot or didn't remember or didn't really pay attention, so it didn't get done.

I do want to lose weight. But that's not the focus of what I'm doing. I'm tracking and using my tools. I'm running trail mix instead of eating it. As I keep being aware of positive changes, I will lose the excess weight. It's happening. Moment by moment-um.

I edited out a lot of entries from the end of September to the middle of October. It could have been because I was busier with my race training, but I think it was because I was writing about a lot of slipups in my eating. I'm noting the time gap, though, because I think it's a red flag to be aware of the importance of food balance for eating and running. I completed my training and ran my half marathon, but my blog posts at this time were a bit of a drag.

POST-HALF MARATHON POST
October 14, 2013

I want to write about my half marathon experience. But I also want to write about the days leading up to the half marathon. The painful knee. The sore calf muscles. Recognizing that although the pain was real, there was a good chance that my brain was using it to distract me from admitting I was nervous and a little scared. And in accepting that, my knee suddenly didn't hurt anymore. I went from having difficulty using stairs to no pain at all.

Last week I ran three and a half miles on Monday. It was about all I could do. I was tired of running. I took the rest of the week off to rest. I walked places, but I did not run. My husband and I went on an overnight trip to Newport, Rhode Island, on Thursday. Friday morning we used the elliptical machines in the hotel gym. I did a mix-up of front and back for a half hour.

Friday afternoon we picked up our race bibs, and my husband bought me a 13.1 T-shirt because he believed I would do it. Nerves set in again, but I was ready for them. Saturday was a beautiful day for my first half marathon. My husband and I waited together for the start. And then, because he was aiming to break two hours, he ran ahead of me. I saw him reach up and touch the starting banner, and then he was gone. I set my Garmin as I crossed the start, and I was running all the way to the finish line. I had a good time. I liked running again.

I chatted with a few other people during the race. It was a friendly atmosphere. I smiled most of the way. And at the finish line, my husband cheered. He had set a new personal record of one hour and fifty-eight minutes, and I had set my first personal record of two hours and forty-two minutes!

We met up with each other at the athletes' food tent. (Yes. I am an athlete!) And then we went to get free massages. My left calf muscle was aching, and the therapist worked both sides. It felt great until I got up to walk again. We made it back to the car. The plan was to go home, shower, and nap. But we ended up skipping the nap and going to get massages. A whole hour from head to toes. Wonderful. My leg didn't hurt quite so bad. And then it did again. Really bad.

I started wondering about a brain/pain distraction thing that I'd read about. I wondered if my brain was latching onto the pain, so I wouldn't deal with some emotion. And I realized I had tried to downplay completing my first a half marathon at age fifty-one. I'd felt like I was tearing up to sob as I crossed the finish line, but I didn't let myself cry. I didn't know if I'd be able to stop. And so I was numb and in a lot of pain.

I replayed the scene in my head and really let myself think about my emotional response to finishing the half marathon. I thought about my resentment of the time it had taken to train (while training). I relived my thrill of actually sticking to a training program and trusting it would carry me to 13.1 miles even though I'd never ever run more than eleven and a half miles at a time. And I acknowledged my frustration of wakening my sugar addiction while I was training—partly because I was using energy gels for fuel.

I must have been interrupted or maybe I ran out of characters to use in my post. But I came back to finish my thoughts.

MIND/BODY DISTRACTION REVISITED
October 14, 2013

We have some friends who work in building construction. They're physically tough and in really good shape. But the guy had terrible back problems that would sideline him for a few days at the beginning of every job. He would get some relief with chiropractic adjustments, but it was always temporary. And then someone gave him a book to read—*Healing Back Pain* by John Sarno, MD. He read the book, and his back pain went away. He didn't have to do special exercises. He just read the book. And then he gave the book to me.

I read the book and was fascinated with the idea of the brain using pain to distract itself from dealing with emotional issues. The initial problem that causes the pain is real, but the brain can make it last longer than it has to. It basically distracts the attention from emotional issues to physical issues. Part of the "cure" is to talk to the brain and let it know you're on to it. The idea is to tell your brain that you really are upset or happy or stressed or weary, and the pain isn't going to distract you from knowing that.

Because I write about my foods and moods, I've connected the idea to eating issues. And I see that eating can be a distraction from emotions too. I think I'm hungry, but I'm really tired. I think I'm hungry, but I'm really disappointed. Or sad. Or happy. Or bored. And when I recognize what is really going on, I can have some water or seltzer or herb tea instead of eating. Or I can read and comment on WW blogs. Or write something instead of eating. When I'm not really hungry, I really just need to be aware of my emotions.

I don't really consider myself an athlete, but I do enjoy running and skiing. They not only keep me in shape, but they also they give me thoughts for blog posts!

OH, SNAP!
October 18, 2013

Moving on from running, ski season is just around the corner. That means The Boston.com Ski & Snowboard Expo is working Facebook with lots of contests and promotions for their upcoming show. I won a two-pack of tickets last year. I had entered to win a snowboard and lessons at Snowmass/Aspen. But I won the tickets to the expo instead. That was okay with me. I really don't care much for snowboarding. (I'd rather be skiing than sitting down on the snow, blocking all the skiers at the top of the hill. Oops. Perhaps I should be nicer than that!)

This year, I'm working the contests again. It's fun. It's a great pep rally for the winter season. And I just found out that I won a prize of a whole case of Snap Supercandy! If I were to eat it all, I think I'd be high enough to not need the chair lift. It's an energy candy—with B vitamins and electrolytes and antioxidants. I actually tried the gum last year, and it was great. But the sugar isn't so great, because with me, I lose my impulse controls, and that doesn't always go so well on a snow-covered mountain. And then there's the crash. No thank you.

One of the contests for the ski show involved writing about your first ski/snowboard experience. My entry talked about my first ski experience at Waterville Valley. It was 1989, and I was a twenty-seven-year-old mother of two. When it came time for dividing up the large group of beginners, we had to ski a couple of turns down to the instructors, who would then put us into very beginners or advanced beginners. I executed two beautiful parallel turns and was told to go to the advanced side until I nearly executed the instructor because I had no idea how to stop! (I was headed straight for him!) I was quickly moved to the very beginners group!

I didn't ski again until I was nearly forty. It was like beginning all over again. This time I kept skiing. Then when I was almost fifty, I lost a lot of weight and experienced skiing in a whole new way. This year I will ski for the first time as a grandmother and a half marathon finisher. One of the beauties of skiing is the newness of each season. I hope to enjoy skiing as a senior in a few years!

Here's the healthy-weight connection. It's a lifelong thing. Experiences and conditions change, but the tools are basically the same even if they are a little more high tech. Making tracks or tracking. The newness of every season or seasoning. Twin tips or sirloin tips. Mont Blanc or Blanc Mange. Powder days or powdered milk. Well, something like that.

I'll keep entering the contests. I'm looking forward to going to the ski show to use my free ticket and to pick up my free candy to give away. But the bigger deal for me is to keep using the tools. I'm blogging my pep talks to myself and anyone who might be interested. I'm sweet-talking instead of eating sweets!

On October 17, 2013, there was a system-wide glitch on the WW site. A lot of blog entries were lost in cyberspace, never to be seen again. At first, I was irritated and annoyed that such a thing could happen, and then I found something else to write about.

YESTERDAY'S GONE
October 18, 2013

Don't start thinking about tomorrow.

Hmmm. That makes me think of a song by a Big Mac. Fleetwood Mac (with credits and thanks to songwriter Christine McVie).

If you wake up and your post is gone
Your tracker's empty—what's goin' on?
Open your eyes and look at today
And try to keep track in a different way

Don't start, thinking about tomorrow
Don't wait, today is right here
It will be better than before
Yesterday's gone, yesterday's gone

Why not think about the present
And not about the things that you resent
If yesterday's record is lost to you
Just think of what today can do

Don't start, thinking about tomorrow
Don't start, today's already here

Opportunity knocks! Let it in the door.
Yesterday's gone, yesterday's gone

All I want is to blog awhile
To write some things that make me smile
I know I believe WW works—it's true
I write to remind me and, maybe, help you.

Don't start, thinking about tomorrow
Track today and be of good cheer
It'll be, better than before
Yesterday's gone, yesterday's gone

Don't you look back, don't binge on a snack

Today is the present, and I am here!

"Could've, would've, should've" carries a connotation of regret, but I had no regrets in this next post.

I COULD HAVE
October 18, 2013

I could have gone off the deep end into a pool of food when I found yesterday's posts had been lost, but I didn't. Even if I had, I've learned how to swim this summer. I know how to get back to where I can feel solid ground under my feet and to make good choices on purpose. I know how to live, not under the power of sugar, but to have control over my impulses. No cravings. On purpose.

I could have gotten upset and stomped my feet, but I didn't. I went to Jazzercise. And then I came home and called tech support. Because this community of support is really important to me.

I also could have tried to rewrite my Thursday post. Well, I did. But it didn't go write or right. So, I faced up to the fact that yesterday's gone, and I started thinking about today. That led me to a rewrite of a famous song.

I could have skipped my WW meeting today. But I went, weighed in, and stayed for the meeting even though my favorite leader had taken the day off. I lost 1.2 pounds, earned two Bravo stars, and showed and told my half marathon finisher's story. I'm still in a little bit of shock myself that I did it. The ladies at the meeting had lots of questions about how long I'd been running. There was a glimmer of hope in a few eyes when I said I'd only started running last year and that I was a reluctant exerciser before that.

I could have thought that the leader looked too tiny to have ever had a weight problem. But I looked at her name tag and found out she had lost 180 pounds. I'm so glad I stayed for the meeting and that she ended the meeting with her story of change. It took her twenty-one months to lose that much weight with WW. She went to her first meeting thinking it wouldn't work. But she made changes and started to lose weight. She showed us her big jeans that were so loose she could easily pull them up with both legs in one pant leg and still have them fit loosely. It didn't happen all at once. They were little changes that led to a big change. She could have missed it, but instead, she did it. Now, she is inspiring others to do it. On purpose.

With all the tracking I was doing, it was no wonder my thoughts turned to trains!

ALL ABOARD TO THiN!
October 21, 2013

WW works when I work it.
This train of thought moves me along.
I track everything that I chew-chew.
I'm going to where I belong!

I seem to be on the scenic route
'Cause it's taken a while to get here.
But I'm seeing the way to stay at my goal
And that has to bring me some cheer.

I've been on a reconnaissance mission
So I know what my goal feels like
But I'm finding I have to get back there by train
Though it's sort of like riding a bike.

Eating like a person that's thin.
What do I think of that?
Well, it is the thing that I really must do
If I really don't want to be fat!

Part of my WW history is going to a meeting in the 1980s and hearing the leader tell about her epiphany. She talked about being in her fridge when she suddenly had a conversation with herself.

"Oh! So you've decided to be a fat person."

"What do you mean? I don't want to be fat!"

"But you're eating like a fat person. If you wanted to be thin, you'd eat like a thin person!"

Lightbulb moment. She put down the food, got out of the fridge, and shut the door.

It's a good story. There are times when I've remembered it a little on the late side. I'd already eaten like I wanted to be fat. But there are many more times I've remembered that story in time to help me think beyond the food to the effects of it.

I'm just a few pounds above my goal range. I've rediscovered that when I'm working the tools the right way, I feel empowered. I feel good about what I'm doing. I'm not dieting. I'm eating like a thin person. Because that's who I am inside. And what's covering that is almost gone!

Some of my thoughts were deep, and some were pretty much on the surface. Once in a while, though, I headed for the skies.

LAX TO NSV
October 29, 2013

I recently thought about losing weight and then getting lax about using the tools. That hit home big time. I've been lax more than once, and although that might sound like I'm relaxed, I'm not. It makes me anxious. And irritated. And stressed. Like I'm pressed for time with connecting flights at a huge airport. LAX maybe?

I've been to Los Angeles International Airport once. It was part of a trip to Guam. We arrived at LAX late because of thunderstorms. We slept for a few hours at a local hotel and then went back to the airport for the continuation of our trip. LAX is a huge airport. It's a hub for a lot of airlines. And it's a means of people making connections and getting to destinations.

I don't know how many people miss their flights or make the wrong connections at the airport. But I know when I'm lax, I don't make the best connections and I usually end up somewhere I don't want to be.

I'm detoxing once again from sugar. That's one thing I have great trouble with when I relax and am lax. I hate the way I feel when sugar is controlling me. But because it is a drug to my system, the call is sweet and seemingly harmless. Until I connect with it. Then I crash. Or I just keep connecting more and more with it until I'm soaring into the plus sizes again.

I had a headache yesterday. I was actually glad I had it, because I knew I was detoxing and regaining control. I relaxed a bit about no eating between meals yesterday. But it was dry-roasted, unsalted peanuts. Not the maple, peanut caramel corn I'd made. I didn't eat any of that. It would have gotten rid of my headache superfast. But I didn't want the muddle it would have caused in my thinking. I didn't want the Benadryl-like dopiness it would have put me in.

I could beat myself up about grazing on peanuts. But that's not the point. I didn't go to my husband's dark chocolate stash. I didn't eat the caramel corn. I didn't eat a bowl of corn pops. I didn't even overdose on fruit. I'm seeing an NSV. (As a reminder, NSV in WW speak is non-scale victory.)

NSV is also the airport code for Noosa, Australia. And what I'm getting out of that is a reference to the book: *Alexander and the Terrible, Horrible, No Good, Very Bad Day.* In the book, Alexander wants to move to Australia because of all the bad things that are going on. Perhaps he knew there was an NSV there. I'm thinking there's a good chance of an NSV in any day if I just look for it. I might be going through LAX, but it can be a gateway to NSV if I make the right connections. I just can't get too stressed and do an about-face into desserts.

Today has had its challenges. But I managed to get through the morning without snacks. Sure, I had my lunch at 11:30, but I'd staved it off ten minutes at a time. I had a cup of tea, a bottle of seltzer, and some water. I emptied the dishwasher, and I put groceries away. I boiled some eggs. And I made it to lunchtime. I didn't go to Australia, but it was NSV!

This afternoon I could feel the sugar calling me. It said, "Oh, you would feel *so* much better if you had something sweet or even a piece of bread." Sure, I'd feel better. Until it wore off, and I needed more and more and more. But this time it wasn't more in charge. It was Maureen in charge.

And when I started feeling lightheaded, I had a planned snack of turkey breast, arugula, whole-grain tortilla, and mustard. Granted, it was a hearty snack. But it was also an NSV.

Not long after that, I had the urge to eat. But because I had just had that snack and tracked it, I was able to talk to myself and say in a convincing manner that I was *not* hungry. Instead of eating, I had a cup of perfect peach herb tea! NSV! I think I've made the connection. I'm on my way.

I kept the travel theme for a few posts.

SALAD FOR BREAKFAST. OR IS IT A LATE SUPPER?
October 31, 2013

This morning I had a salad
Complete with spinach and egg
And now I will answer the question
Before you have to beg.

I woke up feeling quite empty
Fixed hubby breakfast and lunch
Thought what'll I have for my breakfast?
I felt like I needed a bunch!

The spinach was out for the sandwich
Two hard-boiled eggs from the fridge
Lots of good salad veggies
And olive oil—just a smidge!

I chopped it all in small pieces
To take far longer to eat
I had a salad for breakfast
NSV! That was my treat!

And then I looked up the local time
In my new favorite place to "go"
In Noosa, Australia: 9:30 p.m.—
A fairly late supper below.

So, yes, I had salad for breakfast
And some might think it quite strange
But my mind's in the land Down Under

NSV—home off the range!

Perhaps you could call this post "out there"
Or, better yet maybe, "Outback"
But NSV/Noosa on Queensland's coast
Is helping me stay on track!

Some folks might think I am kooka-
Burr(a) I really don't think that I am
I'm typing here on my keyboard
Instead of eating jam.

Too much information on the Internet might have prompted this post!

TMI
October 31, 2013

I'm getting a bit of mileage with the airport codes right now. There isn't too much information on Tumling Tar airport in Nepal (TMI). I have some thoughts about it anyway for my second post today.

Perhaps some might be thinking, "Doesn't she *Ever rest*?"

Yes! That's exactly what I was thinking about. Mountain climbing! From LAX to NSV and on to TMI.

I don't know much about mountain climbing. I've been to Mount Rainier and Mount Washington and Guam. That's kind of like a mountaintop in the Western Pacific Ocean. I've also been to Mount St. Helens (that was a blast!), but I wouldn't call any of it mountain climbing. It was either hiking or riding in a car. Or a jet. Or chairlift. Or gondola.

But real mountain climbing is something else. There are training phases. Altitude acclimatization phases involve trekking to higher altitudes and then back down again to rest before going even higher the next time. Not going too quickly. Understanding limits. Recognizing danger. Rest is important. Fluids are important. Planning is important. Teamwork is important. Fitness is important. Finally, the push to the peak. Scaling the mountain. Going up and back down.

In this whole weight-loss journey, or journey of good health, that I'm on, there are a lot of similarities to mountain climbing. It's a bit upside down, of course. (I'm doing this because I climbed too high on the scale!) And the objective is not to go back to where one started. But still! There are attitude adjustments to make. A little at a time seems to be healthier than too fast on the changes. The scaling part goes up and down with pauses for rest. It's not a straight line, but it's okay because that's how it goes. Teamwork—community—it's what Jean Nidetch, the founder of WW, was doing when she invited people over to talk about losing weight. The WW online community is the cyber version of that. Drinking enough water. Recognizing trigger foods. Recognizing trigger events. Staying away from the abyss. Planning. Tracking. Working on fitness. And the goal is not a time or a number. It's a lifestyle for lifetime.

I paused and considered a pause and found a little poem to help me consider my options.

PAUSE
November 10, 2013

I'd like to take a little time
To pause before a bite.
Is it getting in the way of success
Or helping me be light?

What does the opportunity cost
If I eat a lot or a bit?
Does it take away my options
Or help my clothes still fit?

I had a run of justify posts, and then I thought of blame. I found some things to think about—anything's fair game!

BLAME TO BAM!
November 18, 2013

I've been limping along with my program
Using a crutch or two.
Blaming my problems on sugar
Or stressing on what I can't do.

For the past few days, I've been thinking about the word *blame*, and then I was thinking about what happens when I take the LE out. (Lazy Excuse?) It's BAM. I associate that word with Emeril Lagasse even though I'd never watched him cook before looking it up on YouTube this morning. My impression of the word was getting something done with enthusiasm. And I think the video I watched verified that. Doing it. Bam.

I also noticed that he seemed to be doing a version of aerobics while he was cooking. Moving more. Getting rid of the lazy excuse. Blame: I don't feel like exercising. Bam: I did Jazzercise this morning.

I could blame my sugar addiction for a lot of things. Or I can get rid of my lazy excuses and work with the adaptations I have learned in my journey to BAM! I can get things done and keep moving forward with enthusiasm.

Just like justify, blame gave me a few thoughts to write about.

ANOTHER LOOK AT BLAME TO BAM!
November 21, 2013

At 2:35 this morning, I was awake, and my brain went to this post. Specifically, I was thinking about taking the LE out of blame and making it BAM! I assigned Lazy Excuse to the LE in my first post, but I'm rethinking that. Because the idea of lazy excuse could perpetuate the problems associated with blame.

I'm going to go with Learning Experiences. Every experience—good or bad—can be a learning experience. I have the opportunity to turn each one into a positive to encourage me to move forward with success. The idea of moving forward also tells me to leave something behind. That would be the negative connotations and guilt that sometimes come with a tough experience. Deal with it appropriately and appropriate that to the past. Take the learning experience and move forward.

I think of all of the years I was trapped in my sugar-addiction cycle—not really knowing what it was that seemed to turn every success in my weight-loss efforts into a failure. Even now, slipups that I'm dealing with in my quest to regain and maintain control are learning experiences that, addressed in a positive way, can lead me to BAM! Getting it done with enthusiasm. Or maybe just with hope and confidence.

I've focused quite a bit on what could be seen as bad experiences. But the good experiences also need to be dealt with appropriately. A farmer with a successful crop doesn't keep the plants after the harvest. They get plowed back into the soil to get ready for the next season for more success. And the lessons of the previous seasons help toward the continuation of success.

I can be happy about scale victories and non-scale victories. Celebrate them. But they aren't an ending point. I need to see them as an encouraging point. To keep doing what works. I could mope about my sugar addiction and everything that entails. But that plays right into the addiction cycle. Instead, I can embrace each learning experience (good or bad) and put it in its rightful place so it can encourage me to continue on. BAM!

I wrote about hippo critical earlier, but this was a more academic view.

HiPPO CAMPUS
November 26, 2013

This isn't about the freshmen fifteen. Or even a college for hippos. But I just read an article about sugar and depression anxiety that included a reference to the hippocampus. My title is a twist on that.

I googled "sugar and depression," because I'm feeling a bit concerned about how things are going with my eating and thinking right now. I have a lot of personal experience regarding the effects of sugar on my system. I had a good grip on control for about a year. But the past year, I've been struggling. I've known what to do, but I haven't done it consistently. And in feeling a bit like a broken record, I decided to check into some other sources besides my personal experience and *Potatoes Not Prozac*. Google delivered: "About 42,200,000 results (0.36 seconds)."

Hippo Campus. It's rather appropriate that it's an area of learning and memory. And it's rather scary to think of the effects of sugar or added sugar on my brain. Fuzzy thinking. Impaired memory. And worse. This is way more expensive and costly than any college or university my daughter is considering.

It's not a matter of waiting until after Thanksgiving. Or any other holiday. Or the next morning. This is a quality of life and living thing. I got a grip on it again last evening. I still had a grip on it this morning. It was enough of a grip to say no to leftover salad because it had dried cranberries and maple sugared pecans.

It's not about the weight. That matters, but it's really about my mind. That matters more.

I'm learning. And I'm thankful.

Thanksgiving morning I was thinking about denial and deprivation. And I was thankful to realize that when I indulge in certain things, I'm denying myself of good health and feelings. I decided I wasn't going to deny or deprive myself of enjoyment of family and friends.

CLEANED UP
November 28, 2013

This was the first year my mother didn't do everything about the Thanksgiving meal. My two sisters and I helped plan and cook. Our families helped also. My mother did the turkey, gravy, and stuffing. For the first time in my memory, my dad didn't carve the turkey. He is still recovering from the major stroke he had last May. We were ever so thankful he was with us today at the table.

The meal was fabulous. For having six cooks involved, things went very smoothly. I chose to grill the butternut squash instead of our traditional boiled and mashed. I used a little olive oil and rosemary; sea salt and fresh cracked pepper; and a foil-lined grill. It was amazing. And cleanup was easier than pie!

Turkey; gravy; stuffing (with sausage, onion, and apple); creamed onions; roasted Brussels sprouts with walnut oil; fresh green beans; grilled butternut squash; tossed salad with red onions, gorgonzola, and toasted pecans; homemade spiced cranberry, apple, pear sauce sweetened with maple and honey; rolls; and butter.

I had a little of all of it. Except the rolls and butter. For dessert, I had the leftover salad and veggie sticks.

I skipped the baklava and other Lebanese pastries that one of the guests brought. And I skipped the apple pie and ice cream, pecan cream cheese pie, pumpkin pie, and cranberry orange bread pudding (all homemade). I ate more veggies and hummus (also homemade).

I'm not sure exactly how much I ate today. I do know I did a little grazing with veggies and hummus. And that worries me a little. But I chose to not have sweets. And I'm thankful, very thankful, for that.

The turkey carcass has been boiled and picked. The pots and pans are put away. The kitchen is clean. I feel like I ate clean today. And as a result, I feel clean tonight. Yes, I'm thankful.

I think it's appropriate to find something to be thankful for every day. Even, or especially, on the days that are tough.

REMEMBERING THANKSGIVING
December 2, 2013

I didn't have to worry so much about Thanksgiving or the day after. It's the day after that and today that I wasn't ready for. The big deal is to remember to be thankful. There is much to be thankful for. And it doesn't have to be the fourth Thursday in November to notice it.

I discovered new meanings for words when I looked at them from a different perspective. The definitions aren't found in a dictionary, but they help me understand how to approach certain situations.

DISCOVERY!
December 6, 2013

I've thought of myself as an addict
With a need to continually recover.
Imagine my happy and cheery delight
When I found what I need to discover.

Covering something hides it.
Re-covering hides it once more.
No wonder I'd been on this road many times
To reach goal and fall on the floor.

So in thinking about my journey
With this sugar-sensitive thing
I've uncovered and discovered what I must do
And it makes me want to sing!

Dis-covering something opens it up
And puts it right in plain sight.
The things I must face if I want this to work
To do it and not just I might.

When I re-cover me up with numbers

It sets me up to fail.
I lose sight of good health—my lifetime goal
And gain upon the scale.

Dis-covering (tracking) the finer points
Fit for eating and writing and moving
Helps me to see the ultimate me
And that's what I want to be proving.

Discover connotes a feeling of new
And every day is just that!
I discover the gift of the present—right now!
Dis-cover *me* out from the fat!

Literally or figuratively, I was always looking for a way to keep going.

FiGURATiVELY SPEAKiNG
December 7, 2013

I just logged in my breakfast.
My body already had
But I tracked it on the WW site
And I'll say it made me glad.

I joined to use this set of tools
For quite precisely that
And no wonder when I let it slide
I started getting fat.

The whole idea of healthy
Is way more than just the weight.
It's learning how to deal with things
On literal and figurative plate!

Loading up the literal plate
With lots and lots of food
For me it wrecks my figure
And really spoils my mood.

But dealing with the figurative plate
And the stresses that life piles on
Facing it squarely and treating it fairly
Leads to a battle won.

I liked the idea of calm clarity. Maybe it sounded like a nice, hot drink on a cold day.

CALM CLARITY
December 9, 2013

I got a notification from WW last week. I have until December 21 to weigh in within two pounds of my lifetime goal weight to get another eight-week voucher for free eTools. This is a scary place for me.

I've been aware of it since October. And I haven't been able to keep myself together long enough to lose the weight. In fact, I weigh more now than I did at the end of August. It hasn't been a steady rise. But it's a dreaded yo-yo effect that keeps going higher. I think it's because I'm thinking D.I.E.T (Do It Every Time, aka sabotage). I will say I've had a good week even though I've been sick. Or maybe it's because I've been sick? The sugar detox headache blends in with the sinus pressure. It's all miserable, and I haven't felt like eating much more than soup.

This morning I felt much better. As I fixed myself an egg and toast with a teaspoon of olive oil for breakfast, I realized it was just what I wanted. And when I tracked it, there was a sense of calm clarity that felt right. I have been baking cookies for a funeral luncheon I'll be at tomorrow. Brownie biscotti and oatmeal raisin. Based on history, I know what they taste like. My daughter confirmed they were good. But I know they don't taste better than this sense of calm clarity I feel.

I kept busy this morning and drank toasted coconut créme seltzer as I went about my work. I started feeling hungry just about the time I should eat lunch. I fixed some chicken salad, Jarlsberg cheese, and baby spinach on a whole-grain tortilla and dry grilled in a frying pan atop the stove. I ate a half cup of fat-free plain Greek yogurt and a cup of defrosted mango chunks to finish off my meal. I was satisfied. I tracked my food. And I felt satisfied again, because I'm doing what works for me.

So back to the impending weigh-in. Maybe I should word it a little less ominously. Back to the scheduled check-in at the WW center. This isn't about the numbers. It's about me doing what works for me. Using the WW tools to track my food and moves. Using the blog to track my moods. The weight will come off as a side effect. I've proved it before. And I'm proving it again. With calm clarity.

Something to sync about?

SYNC OR SUNK
December 15, 2013

My husband drives a Ford C-Max. He really likes it, but there have been a few recalls—mostly due to the Ford/Microsoft/Sync My Ride navigation feature. Fortunately, the problems haven't been of Titanic scope, but the "sync my ride" thing makes me laugh. And I wonder if the people who named it ever said it out loud.

It also makes me think of some weight-loss or whole-life things.

The winter season is full of specialty foods that, typically, are available only around the holidays. Lots of sugar. Lots of fat. Lots of triggers. I think about that. And in navigating through the mine (or iceberg) fields of holiday parties, I think having my body tracker (it's automatic and it works *all* of the time) and eTools tracker in sync could be the means of helping me not sink into the abyss of excess food.

Sync is short for *synchronize*, which means in harmony or accord (or in the case of my husband's car, in Ford). There's a sense of order, and perhaps peace, that goes along with the thought. And I think that plays out in using the WW tools. It's not necessarily an easy thing to do all the time. Sometimes there needs to be a recall or reboot. But I know that right now—because I have synchronized my use of the eTools with my rules for dealing with my sugar addiction—I feel a sense of order, even peace, about food.

Yesterday I made two batches of almond toffee (think Brown & Haley Almond Roca). I didn't eat any, and I'm hoping I didn't absorb any of the butter or sugar through my skin when I was shaping the toffee pieces. But I think I'm okay. I know what this candy tastes like (really, really good), but I also know how I feel when I eat it (out of control—as in wanting to eat it all—and then lethargic and dull and disgusted). In taking a moment to see beyond the moment, actually eating this stuff loses appeal. I can remember my mother making it—those are nice, warm-and-fuzzy memories. The memories don't have any negative impact on my tracker. And so I'm fine with just the sight and smell and feel of that candy. No need to taste.

I see something yummy.
Think "How will I feel?"
The answer can cause
It to lose its appeal.

I think this thought, along with the sense of order and control I feel right now, will help me navigate through these next few weeks.

It's hard to avoid sugar. It's a major part of family events. Just because I couldn't handle it didn't mean it wasn't welcome at places I needed to be. I had to get my head around reality and make peace with it.

EXPECTATIONS (A PLAN)
December 19, 2013

I have been asked to make biscotti for Christmas brunch. I've been putting off making it, because I've had a little trouble getting my head around it. Not my mouth, but my head. I think now, however, I have resolved that what I choose to eat is up to me. Whether or not I make the biscotti, people will choose what they will eat. It's up to them. Some people are quite capable of eating one or two, and that's what they do. Just because I don't seem able to stop—even when I feel like I'll pop— doesn't mean I need to hold back on my creative process of making the biscotti. I just have to hold fast to the feeling I have when I'm not under the influence of sugar! My biscotti will not be the only possible temptation available at that brunch. And so, I do not think I need to feel responsible for derailing anyone from an eating plan.

No need for chagrin!
I will not begin!
I'll just savor the sight and the smell.
It won't go to my waist!
Not even a taste!
Or I'll have a dragon to quell!

That feels much better!
I'll fit in my sweater.
And sweeter than that I have found
That if I'm controlling
When sugar's cajoling
I'm happier thin than when round!

I remember being quite resolved to stay in control, and that's what I did. It wasn't easy, but it was worth it.

GETTING RID OF THE GRUMPIES
December 20, 2013

I've been working my tools really hard—logging, jogging, Jazzercising, blogging. I'm trying to get my free pass for eTools by the time it runs out tomorrow. It's been a struggle to stay out of diet mentality, because numbers matter for that pass. Numbers are what have derailed me in the past.

So after having a great week of steady, slow losses on the scale with the prospect of being able to weigh in this morning, the numbers didn't work. And I felt like a jerk. Though there really wasn't reason for that. It's the ugly self-talk. The shame giving walk. That's a part of what leads to fat.

I'm aware that if I were on sugar right now, it would be binge time. Unhinge time. Throw-caution-to-the-wind time. But I'm not on sugar. I'm clean. Even in the midst of baking biscotti and making toffee, I haven't caved to it, and I haven't craved it. I'm not a slave to it. This psychological land mine I'm traipsing through right now is not going to get me.

When I logged in on the WW site to record my breakfast this morning, I saw my friend's status update. She has lost more weight, and she's very close to reaching her one-hundred-pound star. I've been following her story since she started in October 2012. Life hasn't been easy for her, but I'd say it has been better. And she's working the tools. In control. And thinking of her and other success stories in the making, I feel less grumpy. Actually, I'm feeling happy now! Happy to be here. Ready to keep on using the tools!

I have quite a bit of experience with being in control during the holidays only to cave after. This year I was on guard. Not on de fence.

'TWERE THE DAYS AFTER CHRISTMAS
December 28, 2013

'Twere the days after Christmas
And all through the house
Leftovers lurked
To fill out a blouse.

The feasting was tracked
With oh so much care
To keep the scale numbers
From goodness knows where.

The non-scale vict'ries
Were tracked in my head
And the feeling of wellness
Replaced that of dread.

And then … the leftovers
There on the platter
Sent out a pitiful
What—don't I matter?

The cookies, the candy,
The candy canes, truffles
The chips and the snack food
Of Lay's brand or Ruffles.

A snitch that is quicker than
Any old flash
Tells me quite clearly
It belongs in the trash!

The mem'ries of family
Are dearer than food
That clogs up my pipes
And spoils my mood!

And so with kind thoughts
To the labors of love
The leftovers go
With a push and a shove.

The peace that remains
Is full of good cheer
And wishes to all:
Happy Healthy New Year!

And speaking of the New Year …

SELL YOU LiGHT
January 1, 2014

This time of year is famous
For starting a weight-loss journey
And in prior times for me

It looked like a yo-yo tourney.

I'd start on a diet
Really gung ho
Only to crash
With a feeling of woe.

Trying this
And trying that
Wanting a quick fix
To get rid of fat.

Perhaps this fabulous potion
Or some newfangled lotion
A food combination commotion
But not much locomotion.

Maybe a promising DVD
Or sign up with a gym
An advertised wonder—guaranteed.
To make me slimmer than slim!

I'd like to point out that guaranteed
Comes with a few disclaimers.
They refer to diet and exercise
And you have yourself to blamers.

I've found quite clearly in the past two years
That the answer, for me, can't be bought.
Sure there are tools and a few well-placed rules
But I must heed the things I've been taught.

It's not a quick fix from a salesman
With a plan to sell you light.
It's being aware—being able to care—
Support from the blogs—from all, everywhere.
Working the tools in a personal way
Reading comments that oft make my day
People who *know* what I'm trying to say
That detoxing again is more than okay.
It's keeping on going—lifetime at goal
Go On And Live! That's how I roll!

And speaking of rolls, I don't have as many!
My belt doesn't buckle real tight.
And my husband noticed the other day
I have way less cellulite!

Poetry emotion might be a good lead-in to this next post.

COMPASSION
January 3, 2014

We're each on a personal journey
Not marching along in lock step.
Some folks steadily plod along
And others have much more pep.

The stages of learning are varied for all.
Some curves are really quite steep.
To scale them with ease,
Won't you tell me how, please?
I'll listen and not make a peep!

If only that were the answer.
But it wasn't that way for me.
I had to find out with no shadow of doubt
That sugar is poison to me.

It took me long years
To see my way light:
I must control sugar
And do what is write!

I'm not here without any stumbling.
I started and stopped, and I crawled.
And I will not pretend that goal weight is the end.
I thought that a few times and falled!

The tools that I use—they're for lifetime.
I'm learning new things every day.
I continue to work what works well for me.
I'll be here, and that's quite okay!

There's justavacation or justification
For missed steaks and loaded potatoes.

Choices to track or slightly hold back
And maybe pasta tomatoes!

I cannot despise
The road leading to this.
The yo-yo diets.
The feeling amiss.

In learning that diets
Are out of my fashion
I'm learning to live
With much more compassion!

There's an old saying that my husband's grandmother used to quote: "When the days start to lengthen, the cold starts to strengthen." This was certainly true here.

WHIRL WIND
January 7, 2014

The weather pattern right now is called a vortex. That makes me think of a water park ride named that—it looks like a giant toilet. The ride is not something I would go on, but the weather is kind of mandatory. We deal with what we get. That goes along with lifetime. When it's cold, it makes sense to bundle up. When life is rough, there are choices to make that can help or hinder. I guess that's what this post is about.

My dad had a stroke last May. After making quite a bit of progress with recovery, he started to decline again. He was back at home with my mom and extra help, but this past Saturday, it was clear that he needed to be seen for evaluation. With the encouragement of medical professionals, my mom made arrangements for him to go to the hospital. He was admitted, and they are still doing tests to see what is going on. Medical technology is amazing. But sometimes results are not instantaneous. A person (and the whole family) has to be patient!

Since my dad's initial stroke, there have been a few times when I had to make the one-hundred-mile trip while I was tired. Sometimes I would stop at the grocery store for snacks to keep me awake while I was driving. A bag of Skinny Pop. Sure it's only thirty-seven calories a cup, but I'd eat the whole bag of popcorn. The whole family-sized bag. I'd also eat a bag of day-old pastries I'd found (gone looking for) in the back of the store.

I'd get home without falling asleep, but I'd crash after that. I'd wake up with a sugar hangover and need to detox again.

For me, it's not just a matter of saying I'm going to cut back on sugar. I don't have experience with other drugs or alcohol. But I know that sugar as a drug feeds my brain a lot of lies. And it's not an easy thing to regain control once I've lost it. There's a chemical imbalance that I have to work hard to overcome.

So yesterday, when I was starting my ride home, I stopped at a store. I was really tired because I'd stayed overnight in the hospital with my dad on Saturday. Instead of getting junk food, though, I got a chicken wrap (for the chicken), a bottle of toasted coconut créme seltzer (for the hydration), and cut pineapple and a pint of blueberries (for bulk). It was a bigger snack than I usually have, but it was all trackable within my plan. I felt a twinge of temptation to get junk. But I looked beyond the wrapper to the trapper of sugar and what it would do to my brain. (And for some reason, that sentence has triggered a rhyme. It's something I just can't explain!)

I made it home with a stop and stretch at Sam's Club. I was stretching my body and also my dollars. And because I wasn't on sugar, I was able to stick with getting just what I needed. I was still tired, but I was focused and able to function with clarity. The old me saw the loud and tempting ads for cheap food at the front of the store. But the new me, or perhaps I should write, the real me, turned toward the exit and made my way home safely to salmon, red potatoes, snap peas, ginger tea, and bed.

This morning I was given the smallest waist-size lead shield for my mammogram. I'll be patient for the results.

I remember a game that involved clues that could include the phrase "sounds like." I don't remember much else about the game, but that seems to be what my brain was doing with the month.

JANUWARY OR JANUWORRY
January 9, 2014

I wrote a post about this once—I think it had to do with being aware. Perhaps it was about being wary of hurdles that pop up this time of year. Jan. You Wary. Or maybe it's about fretting over resolutions? Jan. You Worry. Or maybe it was a take on a foreign accent—Don't You Worry? I'm going to go with not worrying.

I am helping my folks with my dad's recent hospitalization and move to rehab (last night). He seems to have had another stroke. Maybe some other things are going on. There are a lot of opportunities to worry, but there's also a lot of opportunity to trust.

There's a weight-loss journey (or whole-life journey) analogy here. I could worry about a lot of things, but I am choosing to trust the good-health tools that have worked so well for me. They are adaptable to any life situation. Even hospital and rehab experiences. I'm packing food when I can. And I'm taking my laptop. I'm not eating between meals. I'm checking the blogs. That's one of my tools. Drinking enough water is another. And I'll get some exercise.

I'm very aware of hurdles and snares that abound this time of year. I've gotten through some that have tripped me before. And I'm not thinking because I did that once or twice it means I won't have any more temptations or attempted knockout punches. I am writing, because it is part of the awareness that helps me beware and see where I'm going. So I can make better choices and ultimately wear what I want to because my clothes fit!

My dad is on a bit of a roller coaster with his recovery. And that puts us on one too. But we have trust that all will work together for good. That takes care of the worry. I'm headed into the rehab center now. I'm looking forward to seeing my dear dad. I'll see what I can do to support him and cheer him on as he works this chapter of his life.

To weigh or not to weigh. That was the question.

SKIRTING AN ISSUE. OR NOT.
January 13, 2014

I weighed myself this morning. I was down a pound from the last weigh-in. After I went to Jazzercise, I weighed myself again. Down more. And then on dressing, it seemed like today would be a good day to weigh in at the WW center to get my free eTools voucher and not have to pay for another month. These days have been super busy. I haven't been home much, and it was hard to leave my dad on Saturday afternoon.

My original plans for this week involved heading back to Boston on Tuesday, but with how things seem to be going, I'm planning to go back today. But first, I had to take my daughter to the Minute Clinic to check for strep throat. (No on rapid test, but waiting for the culture for sure.)

Then I paid the tax bill and mailed some packages. My daughter was game to ride with me to my weigh-in, and I was glad for her company.

I went in, used the restroom, and waited for the only other customer to finish up with the receptionist. Then I stepped up to the scale, after I took off my watch and my blazer. I was over my allowable weight by two-tenths of a pound. *Aaargh.*

The receptionist tried to find a way for it to work, but I was already at the top of my range for my height. So she asked me if I wanted her to lock the door and weigh in without my skirt—no one would see! I figured I'd be more covered up than if I were at the beach, and so I said I'd try it.

My skirt was worth four-tenths of a pound. And she gave me my lifetime eTools voucher! I'm back in the ranks of free eTools. To use them wisely. I'm not throwing caution to the wind and figuring I'm done, but I'm continuing to use the tools the way they work for me. Managing my sugar sensitivity. Exercising. Blogging. Tracking.

My dad's health continues to decline. The goal is to keep him comfortable right now. My mother and sister are with him. And I will be heading there again soon. It's a sad time for our family. A reminder that our bodies are not designed to last forever. We do what we can while we can. Our faith helps us see beyond the moment and trust for the soul that continues on.

It may seem frivolous that I took time to weigh in today. But I am thinking it was fitting. And my dad will or would be pleased to know that I'm back to free. With his love and support.

Can I afford to put in another reference to my husband's car? I'll try it.

POINTING THE WAY?
January 14, 2014

Yesterday, when I was going to the rehab place where my dad is, I tried to enter the location into the navigation system. I was driving my husband's C-Max, and it has voice-activated controls. I had difficulty making myself understood to the system. I think I have clear diction. I was born in Boston, but my mother is from the West Coast and my accent is fairly dictionary-like. Perhaps I should have tried the Boston accent. Nothing I said came up with the destination I wanted.

I finally came up with what I thought was the name of the facility. The street name was different from the address of the rehab center, but it was the name of the side street the entrance is on. So I put that as my destination. I wasn't thinking about the possibility that a large city could have multiple streets with the same name.

My dad wasn't doing well. My mom and youngest sister were already there. My older sister was on her way from a different direction. And I was going to arrive a little later than originally planned because of my decision to weigh in at WW for my free eTools. When I made the turn onto what I thought should have been the side street to the facility, I could see that it was actually a defunct rehab laundry center on a dead-end street that was in a different section of Boston. Not only did my ride sink, my heart did too.

I got to the right place in time. But the ride there was through some interesting neighborhoods—ranging from ultranice to not so nice. I got there by putting in a different point of interest that I knew was near where I wanted to go. It worked, but I ended up using a lot of time and energy that could have been used for something else had I just taken the time to make sure I was headed to where I really wanted to go.

I'm seeing my weight-loss journey in this story. I've set out many times to be healthier. But most of the time I found I was using the wrong directions. It wasn't really until I got to a dead-end street and feeling really lost that I found directions to a place nearby—a place of controlled sugar intake—that I was able to get to my healthy range of weight. In reducing my sugar consumption, keeping my eating to mealtimes, tracking my foods and moods, and moving more, I found the way to mental clarity and my healthy-weight range.

My dad was much better today than he was yesterday. There are renewed feelings of possibilities. And each day will be as it is. Today I ate three meals that I tracked. I made countless runs to the kitchen for ice cream or drinks for my dad and mom. All this and more while I was on the phone trying to help my eighteen-year-old daughter through her sore throat/ear pain that turned into her first solo visit to a clinic for ear infection diagnosis and meds. And when I got back to my folks for the night, I ran my fastest treadmill mile ever.

I have been on an emotional roller-coaster ride. But my food is logged. My mood is blogged. My mile is jogged.

I'm sure I was referring to the fifteenth of the month in this post. I just twisted it a bit for my purposes.

I'DS OF JANUARY REVISITED
January 16, 2014

Yesterday was a busy day. Again. I was at the rehab place with my dad and mom for the morning, and then I headed back home to the generation on the other side of me. I'm working a balance to stay healthy, and I'm glad to say that my fuel for the trip home was a healthy, balanced snack of protein, fruit, and black coffee. The popcorn, muffins, and candy of prior trips were available to buy, but they didn't appeal to me because I didn't want the effects they cause. It feels like an ongoing victory that's helping me get and be where I need to be.

The roller coaster continues as far as my dad's condition goes. But there is a sense of appreciation for what is unfolding with strength to keep going. Things were a bit low yesterday, but then there was an upturn this morning. Again. It's impossible to know if he will rally and be able to go home again soon. Or if his time with us is nearly over. We don't even know that about ourselves. Someone said to my mother yesterday that death isn't a medical procedure, but a life event. It isn't a failure. It is part of life. It's a helpful thought. And it went along with some thoughts that have been working in my head and heart.

This is a time of doing what we can. While we can. Showing love and support. Feeling love and support. Moving forward in the right direction. We can't quite see the future. But we trust it will be right.

Though it might seem rather trivial in comparison, there are some analogies back and forth with the WW process and lifestyle. And I'm thankful.

The phrase "I'd have" many times is followed by a *but*. Often, it's a big but. Sometimes, the but is helpful. I'd have bought a big bag of popcorn and some day-old muffins to help me stay awake on the ride home yesterday, but I didn't want to experience the negative consequences that sugar and between-meal grazing always leave behind (which sounds like bigger but). This kind of I'd/but is helpful.

I'd have started eating healthy and all that, but I had a lot of leftovers to use up and the Christmas candy was on sale for 90 percent off. I reasoned this way a lot for years. That kind of I'd/but leads to a bigger one, and that's not very helpful. I suppose one could say that's the backside of that phrase.

So here, on the day after the ides of January, I'm thankful for many things. I'm thankful to be working my tools and not standing by I'dly with a big but.

As life for me went on, it was clear that my father's life would be ending soon. If there were a list of emotional experiences, this would be at the top. I found it to be reasonable and prudent to keep using my tools.

WAIT WATCHING
January 17, 2014

Today was another day waiting to see what will happen. Watching. The journey of life continues another day. I continue to eat three meals a day with restricted sugar. I'm working a careful balance of protein and carbohydrates and regular hydrates. I'm exercising and waiting until mealtimes. I'm watching to be aware of how I feel.

This evening I chose to eat a Reuben sandwich. It appealed to me, and I tracked it. I was full and satisfied and maybe a little more than that. I noticed. I won't be having another one really soon, but that's okay. I can wait. And watch for the right time if it happens to come.

I never realized how much energy this wait watching can consume, and yet, I feel like I need to expend more energy with physical exercise. There's a certain release in moving, and I'm glad for some minutes on the treadmill.

I think in this situation of so many things being outside of my control, the things that I can control are feeling good. Choosing to wait. And remembering to watch. For lifetime to go on.

I'm writing another overtired post, but it's my way of working through some things toward sleep and toward waiting and watching for the new day. The new week. The new opportunities. And so on.

When it came time for only comfort measures in my dad's care, there was a certain resignation that came with it. But there was comfort for us too in doing what we could.

COMFORT MEASURES
January 18, 2014

We are in the comfort-measures stage. It is not an easy time, but there are comforts in spending time and being with family. It's a soft time. But it's not because I have extra padding on me. This afternoon I noticed I was able to properly snap the snow skirt on my ski jacket and not have to leave one set of snaps undone.

Comfort measures for me have been taking care of what is most important to me and working on maintaining my health. I went for a run this morning before driving my mother to the rehab. I had breakfast, lunch, and supper. I had a planned snack of two cheese sticks and a banana. I tracked it all. My run is tracked along with the hour of snow shoveling. It was heavy, wet snow in wonderfully cold air. I welcomed exercise after being inside for so long.

There are lots of food options around. Some are healthy, and some are not. I find comfort in sticking to my three meals and a planned snack. I find comfort in staying away from sugar so I can be present in this experience, because even though there is much sorrow in the thought of my dad not being here soon, there is much joy in the thoughts of his life and love. What he has lived for makes this time not scary but the next step for him. Death is not a failure but a life event. And in being prepared for it, there will be a sense of victory.

Comfort measures. There are so many things that are out of my control. I'm finding comfort in taking care of the things that I can control. I know my dad would be proud.

This afternoon, I had planned to head back home for a couple of days. But then I realized I would miss out on precious time with my dad and mom and sisters. The things I thought I had to take care of would wait. My husband lovingly supported my decision to stay a little longer. Fortunately, my youngest daughter has no school on Monday. We, along with my oldest daughter, rode together to the rehab center this evening where we shared supper and stories and silence and solace and even some silliness together. Comfort measures.

And with that, I'll just add that there is a bit of added comfort in the WW program when a person measures and tracks accurately. The body and the tracker agree, and there are fewer surprises at the scale. And even if there is a surprise at the scale, there is comfort in knowing the tools will work as I work them.

The end came, but there was a continuing that went along with it.

LiFE'S JOURNEY
January 19, 2014

This poem is not about weight loss or weight maintaining. It is very personal. Yet, I feel like sharing.

There comes a time in the journey of life
When the body is no longer needed.
The soul leaves an empty shell behind
For a call that must be heeded.

So sweet when that call
Is the voice of a Friend
Known well in lifetime
And true through the end.

Right now we continue
To fill a place
Of support with support
And loving grace.

Thankful for life
For its joys and its sorrows
If today is the last
Or with many tomorrows.

At some point the ties
To this life will be broken
The love is strong
Felt—if not spoken.

My heart overflows through my eyes with tears
Expressing what I cannot say.
I'm thankful for faith and a living hope
That provision's been made for this day.

I'll miss the grip of Dad's loving hand
And his way of expressiveness

But I'll rest assured with a comforting thought:
Right was the pathway that led up to this.

*During this experience, I was blogging as part of my control over
sugar. I found an outpouring of support from my online WW friends
in the comments they'd post after my blog entries. I knew I had people
thinking of me with sympathy and care. I also knew they were cheering
me on in my quest to be healthy. It was a big help.*

REALITY
January 19, 2014

My father passed away this afternoon. He was an amazing man, and his
influence will continue with us. His memory will live in many hearts with
a feeling of gratitude and love. There is a quiet strength and comfort.
A sense of peace. A feeling of victory. And oh so much to think about
and do without being bogged down by sugar. My dad had a role in me
staying in control. And I am so thankful.

*Prior to this, I had a vague idea that there were things to do between
death and a funeral, but the reality was much bigger than I'd ever
imagined. I realized, though, that continuing to write would help me be
able to think more clearly. I think it was a little gift for my thoughts to
come out in rhyme this time.*

MACROS WITH EASE VS.
MACARONI AND CHEESE
January 20, 2014

Just a little something tonight.
Blogging is one of my macros
A routine of sorts to stay in control
Instead of eating some tacos.

In changing times (in prose or rhymes)
There are some things that stay the same.
Eating three meals with protein it feels
Like I'm still in and winning the game.

Sugar's not welcome.
Quite matter of fact.
I've learned to say no

With control and tact.

In times that I used to
Seek comfort in food
I now know routines
Can help with my mood.

My mother has, for as long as I can remember, had routines. I didn't always appreciate this, but in the past months I've noticed them more. Because of her routines, she has been able to keep up with her house and health and more while being primary caregiver for my dad.

She has been a Weight Watcher since the 1970s. And she has always looked great. Some people have questioned her being a Weight Watcher. She doesn't look like she needs to lose weight, because she doesn't need to lose weight. She lost her initial amount by developing macros, or routines, with her planning and shopping and eating. She's not on a robotic schedule, and she's not an unimaginative cook. But she has routines, and they have helped her keep her weight where it should be. The tools work for her and continue to work.

My dad was a lifetime Weight Watcher too. His tools were mostly eating what my mom fixed for him. That was his macro for weight control. He had plenty of other routines too. And then the stroke took almost all of that away. At times, the only thing that he could do was to show my mother love and appreciation for all she was doing. And that was firmly in place. Not as a mindless routine, but as part of his being.

I'm working on my macros. Some of them I have firmly established, so I can do the macros with ease. Tracking. Steering clear of sugar. Exercising. And knowing the comfort of having things in order. Yes. I'll take those macros with ease. Instead of seeking comfort in a bowl of macaroni and cheese.

Growing up in New England, I remember some winters with snow and others with not so much. This was one of the winters with snow. Lots of it.

WiNTER ACTiViTY
January 22, 2014

I'm still at my mother's home. The funeral arrangements are coming together. Family will be arriving from afar tomorrow. We had a snowstorm yesterday. And because I didn't have winter boots with me, I used a pair of my dad's. His feet were much bigger than mine, but with fleece-lined tights and my running socks and the laces pulled tight, they worked just fine.

I've never walked a mile in his shoes
But I just shoveled snow in Dad's boots.
Remembering the times when I shoveled with him
Feeling quite close to my roots.

Roots that are grounded firmly in love
Part of our family tree.
Feeling support though he's physically gone
Glad for each sweet memory.

I found it a helpful exercise to think about how things related to my personal growth.

DASHING ABOUT
January 23, 2014

Funeral planning and preparation is more involved than I ever realized. But perhaps it is fitting to be dashing about remembering my dad and getting things done. Someone has written eloquently about the dash between the years of birth and death. My dad's dash was between 1933 and 2014, and I'm thinking that some of that dash was about planning and preparing and doing. I think it's called living.

I am continuing to value the things I have learned to do with WW tools and *Potatoes Not Prozac* guidelines. I have been dashing about with purpose and productivity. I haven't been wallowing in sugar.

There is plenty of sugar around. Thoughtful folks have brought meals and desserts and more. But Maureen is only experiencing them in the sight and smell and intent of kindness. I am fiercely protecting myself and my ability to get through this time as me. There are memories to enjoy. And, yes, pain to feel. It's not easy to say good-bye to a loved dad.

I am here. Taking a little break. Recording my mood. In control of my food. And thankful that I can be a part of a wonderful family with wonderful friends and wonderful support systems.

My mind has a hard time seeing the word fun in funeral. It doesn't seem to fit. I didn't write the dictionary, but I did write how I felt about my experience with my dad's funeral.

WHAT A WEEK
January 26, 2014

Seven days. Seven strong days. Not because I felt able. But because I had so much help on so many levels.

Last Sunday, my father died. And today is the day after his funeral.

I have been present for it all. I did not miss out on the joy and sorrow interwoven that marked my dad's release from the debilitating effects of a second stroke and the separation we feel so keenly because he is not physically here anymore. I feel great comfort in knowing he lived to be ready for this. I have been able to appreciate the support and comfort of so many who were also feeling the loss. I have not buried my sorrows in sugar, because that would have added to my sorrow.

I am tired. But I'm not too tired to be thankful for an experience that was filled with love and care and compassion and comfort.

I have blogged through most of it. And eaten appropriately through all of it. I haven't been able to weigh and measure or even track everything. But I've been able to keep my eating to mealtimes. I've had extremely limited sugar. I ran on the treadmill when I could. And ran up and down the stairs countless times.

I am very aware that awareness will be key in these days that follow. That they also need to be strong days. Not weak days.

When I was putting some sweets away this evening, I had a fleeting thought of sampling them. But I knew the avalanche it could trigger. And on second thought, I was repulsed by the memory of how it has made me feel in the past and what sugar has robbed me of when it has been in control. When I thought of that, it was easy to leave it alone.

This past year, I've let sugar in a few times, and it wasn't pretty. It doesn't take much of a slip to have it take over. But I've gotten better at realizing what is wrong. And although it's not very easy to regain control once I've lost it, I've proved that I can. And I have. With much appreciated help.

I lost a little more than five pounds this week. And that's not a loss I mourn.

I know I continued to be busy with funeral things for a few days, but there came a time when that too ended.

HOME
January 29, 2014

I physically returned to my legal residence yesterday after being away almost two weeks. I went to Boston on January 16 for my father's last days of life. I stayed there through the planning and preparation and funeral services. I was away until yesterday. And now, I am back at my house. Home.

The funeral was Saturday. The last of the out-of-town family left my mother's house on Monday. On Tuesday, I did a little more to put things back where they belonged. And then I drove back home.

I came home to take my youngest to a dentist appointment and to do a Sam's Club shopping trip. My husband encouraged me to go to Jazzercise class last night if I was back in time. I was. I hadn't been able to go for a few weeks, and it was good to move in a class setting with instructions on what to do next. Not too much thinking but a lot of moving.

I'm getting reacquainted with my kitchen and the laundry and some other routine home things. My husband and youngest daughter had kept the place neat while I was gone. (They were with me several times during the time I was away from home, but they had to be back and forth a bit.) This morning I started laundry and decided to go to the morning Jazzercise class—my regular class time. Home again.

But in thinking about it, I've had a sense of being home the whole time I was away. I continued to use my tools. I was checking in online to write blog posts. I was tracking my food and recording treadmill runs. I was reading comments of support and sympathy while trying to read a few other bloggers' posts and write encouraging comments. I've stayed away from sugar and kept close to the comforts of a non-sugar-hazed home. Present even when it hurt. Because it meant more to me to feel the feelings than to be numb and then resurface with a sugar hangover.

I've proven that the way that I use the WW tools to work for me is not a diet but a lifetime aid. The day that I went to Boston, I had weighed in and gotten a new eight-week voucher for free eTools. I was in my goal range. And I got to tell my dad that I'd done it. I didn't throw caution to the wind and use that pass for out-of-control eating. (It's amazing how many sweets were available to eat.) I just continued to use my tools. Enough protein. No in-between-meal eating. A multivitamin. Exercise. And I lost more weight to get me closer to my heart goal weight. It's the weight that fits me better. The weight that makes me feel more at home wherever I am.

Home. Where my heart is.

Part of what comes after a loss is remembering the past and looking to the future.

PULLING WEEDS
January 30, 2014

My nephew told us on Sunday that my dad had taught him how to pull weeds out of the lawn. They had headed across the yard one day, and my dad stopped to pull a piece of crabgrass. He said that the easiest time to take care of weeds was when they were small. And so on the day after his beloved Grampy's funeral, he was telling us about that lesson he'd learned. He related it to natural and spiritual issues. And said he'd like to take care of problems when they're small—before they spread into bigger problems complete with seeds to spread the problem further. Good lesson.

It applies to weight management as well. My mother told me a long time ago that she had learned to respect a pound in either direction. Slow and steady losses are not to be despised. They lead to a goal. Slow and steady gains are not to be trivialized. They lead away from a goal. If gains are not paid attention to, the goal can become more distant than ever before. She's been maintaining her lifetime status with WW for years.

I've been pulling weeds—Weight Watching weeds—lately. I've been nipping bad habits in the thought stage. Thinking beyond the moment to the reality of after. And in the process of doing that, I've gotten back to being able to wear the clothes I bought when I reactivated my lifetime status in October 2012.

2013 was a year with a few too many weeds working their way into my eating habits. By the time I really noticed the damage they were doing, I had gained thirty pounds over my lowest weight. That's twenty pounds above my WW goal weight. Fortunately, I was able to whack the weeds and start pulling them out by the roots. In the process of time and tenacity, I lost the weight as I regained my turf in the world of control.

Yesterday, I wore a beautiful Pendleton straight skirt. Size eight. Today, I pulled a Ralph Lauren skirt, size six, out of my closet. Put it on. Zipped it up. And it fit. No weeds. (I suppose it would have been fitting if the material was Lawn Cloth, but it was denim.)

I'm not going to pretend that weeds won't try to come back. Or that I don't have to think about pulling them ever again. I've done that, and it doesn't work. My clothes don't fit over those weeds. And my mind has a hard time seeing through those weeds. So I'm planning to notice. I'm going to pay attention. I'm going to be aware as I'm walking across my days. And I'm going to yank those weeds out as soon as they think of appearing.

I felt, at times, like I would write a post of realization and determination only to find a few days later that a seed thought from the post would seem to blossom into a huge challenge.

IRRATIONAL NUMBERS
February 4, 2014

I'm not sure where this post is going to go, but I'm here with it. I was dealing with numbers that were completely irrational yesterday. No way to express them in a fraction. No mental clarity or reason to them. I guess I could chalk it up to emotional distress. That would work.

In the recent focus on family tree, the idea of roots comes to mind. I'll call yesterday the square root of two. It didn't make a lot of sense in math class. And it doesn't make a lot of sense here. Irrational. Because that's how it is described. I see it as a placeholder of sorts. And it got me to an answer this morning: I'm human.

In blogging about my experience with using the lifetime WW tools during my dad's final hospitalization, his death, planning the funeral, and experiencing the whole thing without sugar, I got a lot of support and cheering about how well I was doing. The experience of staying in control and being present for it all without the haze of sugar was amazing.

But yesterday I let sugar in. It may have been a gradual thing over the course of the weekend. A lengthening of mealtimes that turned into grazing. Feeling like a sad little girl who misses her daddy, even though I'm fifty-one and a grown-up of sorts. Wanting to escape, in a way, the reality of life and death even though I have seen great beauty in both. Perhaps it was an irrational feeling that tried to convince me it was wrong to have had such strength in such a time as now. To have lost weight instead of gained as I had in the past. To have garnered praise for my strength in staying on plan when the focus should not have been on me.

I think it was a combination of things that started slowly. But yesterday the floodgates opened, and I felt like I was drowning. Except I didn't. Because even in the uncontrolled numbers of points and pounds of irrationality, I could feel the sham of sugar. I was aware that there was no comfort and no real escape.

But really, no *need* to escape. Reality, even with pain, was better, and sugar was bitter. And in seeing that, there's a healing feeling that keeps that sham from turning into shame. It happened. I've put a plan in place for recovery. Because, in looking at what I chose for breakfast this morning, that's where I was. Cooked oats, fat-free plain Greek yogurt, mango chunks. A multivitamin. And water. I didn't measure it. But that's okay. I didn't need to be ration-al about it. Just simply full of good foods and thanks.

Stages make me think dramatic productions, and grieving started living up to that thought.

STAGES
February 5, 2014

Stages of grief. I'm going to work through them as they come. Not as a textbook thing, but as a part of this race I'm in. The human race.

If diving into sugar was part of the denial stage, I'm feeling like I'm ready to move on from the drama it causes. But not too fast. Not "to fast." I'm not going to deny myself of eating right. I'm starting with breakfast. And tracking. Good, clean foods and a slice of homemade oatmeal bread with one teaspoon butter. I'm waiting until lunch to eat again. I'm reading and commenting on blogs. I'm moving. I'm being patient. It's so I can be healthy.

I know from life experience that it doesn't pay to rush through stages. Rushing birthing breathing doesn't speed up labor and delivery. It wears the mother out and confuses the support team. I'm thinking this can hold true for grieving too.

Weight loss and weight maintaining. It's a step at a time in the right direction. On the right stage. And if the first step on the first stage is denial, it's still a step in the right direction. A step to move on from at the right time. To the next stage.

Solid progress on a firm foundation. There's great beauty in it. I can see it now.

When my thoughts came out in rhyme, I felt like I was tapping into a deeper place of thought. As I went back to really read what I'd typed, I'd find helpful hints of what to do.

SHE WHO HESITATES
February 9, 2014

She who hesitates has gained
A tiny bit of wait.
Just enough time to think again—
A helpful weight-loss trait!

I gain so much when I count the cost
Of a mouthful or morsel or bite.
And lose the thought of eat right now
That makes the clothes grow tight.

The wisdom in the second thought
The time it takes to do what I ought
To win the battle that must be fought
Over sugar's wiles and what it has wrought.

There's full-scale value
In counting the cost.
For she who hesitates enough
Can find that she has lost!

I haven't included a lot of information about my weight-loss (and -gain) numbers. I think part of the reason for this omission is because the "shrinking" work I was doing in my mind seemed weightier. But my body weight mattered in obtaining free eTools, and I didn't want to shrink from this bargain!

BLING IT ON!
February 12, 2014

I just got back from my February weigh-in. I have my new free lifetime eTools voucher, a new keychain with a bunch of charms, and a loss in my book. The six-tenths of a pound loss was from what the official scale showed the last time I weighed in on January 13, 2014. There's a bigger story, though, that includes an almost nine-pound gain last week due to an out-of-control sugar problem I was having on my return home from a pretty stressful situation. I had stayed in control marvelously through the end of my father's life, as well as his funeral planning, services, and post-burial luncheon. I had stayed in control for another couple of days until a couple of days after I returned home.

The week before the almost nine-pound gain was a two-pound gain. But the week before that was a 5.2-pound loss. That's how in control I was in the midst of casseroles and sweets and stress. But then, I succumbed to sugar, and the climb out wasn't working. I'll spare the details. But it was changing my attire. I couldn't wear some of my clothes, because I had a spare tire around my middle!

Last week I was not struggling with sugar. Well, actually, it had me wrapped in its tentacles, and I was thinking it was a hug for a little while. But then, as I was gaining weight by the seconds (and thirds), I began to think about my free eTools. And February's weigh-in for lifetime.

My sugar-addicted brain was screaming, "*No! It's only the second week in February! You don't have to weigh in until the absolutely last day of the month!*" The real me quietly decided to take action anyway.

Since Sunday, my weight has been dropping. And today, not even two weeks into the month, I was able to weigh in at the WW center and get my free eTools, because I was in my healthy range. And I had all my clothes on.

To explain my "bling" title: the receptionist was awesome enough to ask some questions about why I didn't have all the WW keychain rewards. She added my online starting numbers to my meeting notes, and I left with a bunch of charms.

My husband and I went on a ski trip. We found some powder and some things to blog about!

POLiSHiNG THE SKiS
February 17, 2014

I realized there was a huge WW connection in my ski lesson about carving. The technique that I was working on involved leading with the head. I was stretching out over the ski in the direction I wanted to turn. The difference that made in my skiing experience was noticeable. The snow was deep and bunched up all over the place. Skiing on the flats of my skis made me feel like I was constantly crossing the wake in waterskiing. It was wearing me out and making me nervous. (I hate to fall.) When I actually used the edges of the skis the way they are meant to be used, I carved through the snow with ease. It was fun and enjoyable. It was exhilarating! Considering the skis are part of the tools I use, using them effectively for the conditions I was in made all the difference!

I'm working my WW tools with the thought of being healthy. Those are the conditions. I'm working with anti-inflammatory foods. I'm not grazing between meals. I'm drinking lots of water. I'm taking a probiotic and a multivitamin. It hasn't been hard. I wouldn't call it fun, but my meals have been good and satisfying. I'm also continuing to lose weight. There is a sense of exhilaration in fitting easily into my thin clothes! I'm seeing this anti-inflammation thing as making sense to my brain. I'm leading with my head. It feels good.

Now to change gears and address my statement of hating to fall when I'm skiing. Since losing a bunch of weight and getting more fit, I am now able to stand up without removing my skis. It has to do with having less to haul up off the ground, and it also has to do with stronger muscles in my legs and my core.

In my past attempts at weight loss and maintaining, I had an all-or-nothing attitude. Follow the rules to the letter and at the first fall, give up and give in and get fat again. I've proven over the past year that I didn't give up. Even when my weight went up, I was able to get back up without taking my skis (tools) off. I think this is because I've been regularly exercising the tools. I'm stronger. I'm more aware of what's going on inside. And I am more aware of what I have to do to keep going.

Falling on skis can happen at full tilt or when I'm hardly moving at all. A fall can be from catching an edge or tripping on a pole. A little off balance. A patch of ice. Or a heap of powder. Hopefully, the fall doesn't cause an injury. But there are tools for that too. If it's just a fall, and that's all, get back up and stand tall! Lean in. Lead with the head. And turn again.

Falling using WW tools and my sugar-addiction guidelines can happen at full tilt or when all seems calm and serene. It happens when I'm not catching enough sleep. Or there are unplanned events. Stress. A patch of ice cream. Or a heap of powdered sugar donuts. The big deal is to get back up. And remember the purpose of the tools. They're to aid in living and playing and working. Making it a little easier. Fun. Enjoyable. Even exhilarating!

I found comfort in food for thought.

COMFORT
March 3, 2014

On my way to the store today, I passed a restaurant with a sign advertising comfort food. I was feeling hungry, but the comfort food I had in mind was more in line with anti-inflammatory foods. I was interested in the comfort of eating what I know is good for me. The comfort of good health. The comfort of eating to stay in my lifetime goal range. Somehow, I didn't think that restaurant was on the same page for comfort food.

That got me to think about comfort food, though. My prior definition of comfort food was high sugar, high fat, high calorie, and high volume. It was false comfort, because even if there was a good feeling while I ate it, there was a bad feeling after. A feeling of lost control. A feeling of wanting more even if my clothes were already feeling too tight.

What changed the definition of comfort food for me was *Potatoes Not Prozac*. It opened my eyes to what sugar does to my brain—erosion of impulse controls, reduced mental clarity, depression, mood swings. And what, in turn, it did to my body—obesity.

As I reflected on my history of change, I realized there was another way to see the word *comfort*. Com For T. Come for tea. This winter has been a time for me to give comfort and also to receive comfort. The idea of inviting a friend in for a cup of tea and a chat has a sense of comfort along with it. And if there isn't a friend available in person, I can choose from a wonderful number of friends in the blogging community. I can read lovely comments on my wall or at the end of my blog posts. I can write little notes to my friends. I can do all of this while sipping a cup of tea. There's a sense of comfort in community.

Come for tea.

LIFETIME: A DAY AT A TIME, SOMETIMES IN RHYME

Listen to Reason: A New Paradigm!

Life goes on. It wasn't a matter of getting my sugar addiction fixed. It was about getting a new paradigm so I could manage my sugar addiction instead of it managing me. I didn't go to the prose, here.

EASY AS PIE? (DON'T I WISH, WITH A SIGH.)
March 13, 2014

Would that it could be so easy
To get out of a sugar pig sty
By writing a poem
Or reading a tome
Titled "It's as Easy as Pie."

(I envision this book
could be *Quiche and Tell*
All of the tricks in
Sugar's strong spell.)

But it's not quite that easy.
For me, I get queasy
And shaky in days two through five.
I stumble and bumble and sometimes I fumble
Working to keep it alive.

Yes, it is work.
But not really a drudge
And it's worth it to me
To get off the pudge.

Not only the pudge,
But the feeling of sludge

Messing up my thought.
So I'm on the train tracking
What I chew-chew and yakking.
Doing the things that I ought.

I'm coming back brighter
Working toward lighter
I've once again paid sugar's toll.
I want to be healthy
In wisdom, be wealthy
To keep going on with my goal.

I suppose some people could keep their money in the deep freeze, but I was more interested in the sugar.

COLD CACHE
March 18, 2014

I used to put things in the freezer
A fairly safe place to hide
Sweets or treats or something to save
For guests from far and wide.

But addiction's powerful cravings
Can bite things as hard as steel
Frozen brownies were tastier
Instead of losing appeal.

So it wasn't a very good hiding place
Because when I needed the stuff
It wouldn't be there 'cause I'd eaten it all
Like I just couldn't get enough.

The scenario I rhymed about happened more than once. Fairly early on in life, I discovered my mother's cold cache of frozen applesauce cupcakes with browned butter frosting, the Ravine Brownies that were more like fudge and the Whitman's Samplers generously given to my dad by his customers.

It's not a great memory. The stuff was good, but the out-of-control feeling wasn't. I had a reputation for getting into sweets. Most of the time when something had been eaten before it could be served, there was a good chance I was involved. But one time, it wasn't me. A mouse got into some Planters' Peanut Bars my mother had bought for trick-or-treaters. It left some calling cards. The real proof that I hadn't snitched from the stash is that there were leftovers.

What I seemed to need back with the freezer and sweets was a little restraint. But it's hard to have restraint when sugar has disabled impulse controls. Addiction has a power that is scary. I've proved it many times.

I've also proved that I can be in control as long as I don't graze between meals and I stay away from sugar. Blogging helps me with my reality checks. I take stock and move forward, making adjustments as needed. Planning for the future. Staying in control. Or reclaiming control.

I think I'm fairly mellow, but sometimes the drama kicks in.

DRAMA MINE
May 8, 2014

The drama of my life right now
Is something I must own.
I'm sick and feeling yucky
And kind of all alone.

My throat is sore
I have a cough
I have fallen
In a feeding trough.

My face is swollen
My glands are tender
Why would I choose
A sugar bender?

This drama mine—emotion sick
With waves of grief and crying
I need to stop and get a grip—
Remember why I'm trying.

This may sound more dramatic than it actually is. I have a cold. And yes, I'm feeling sad. I miss my dad. This week I went to help my mother with yard work. I did it a lot last year when my dad was trying to recover from his stroke. This was the first time I went to do yard work since he passed away in January. The stroke was at the end of last May.

Tuesday I did some final prep for mulching. And then I spread mulch. I figured out how to use the rototiller and turned over the garden. These are things he was doing this time last year. The yard looked like a park before he got sick. And after he was sick, several of us tried to keep it looking like a park.

I enjoyed doing the work. I had lots of good memories to think about. Techniques to use that I'd picked up from watching my dad work. And when I was done, it looked good. But I also really missed him. I wouldn't wish him back to suffer more with the effects of the stroke. But I really, really missed him.

Yesterday, I helped my mother dig out some space for planting flowers at my family's grave site. My dad's name and dates are on the stone now. And my mother's name is there too. With her birth year. She's very much alive, but that's how it's done.

So yes. I'm feeling kind of sad. And a bit bad. I wish I didn't feel so wrong when I choose food that doesn't work for me. (That terrible feeling is what gets me to want to be back on track, though.) I think I was just eating to match my mood. It wasn't a good idea. Because I have to get out of it. Again. I think the grief could be more effective if I let it happen without the food grief too.

I'm reaching for
That happy thought
That can't be bought
The priceless thankfulness
I can and will feel better soon
And not wallow in a mess.

Thankfulness. That's my lifeline. That's what I can hold on to and slowly pull out of the place I'm in right now. I'm also taking Wellness Formula, Claritin, and lots of liquids for my cold and allergies. As far as getting back to normal, this is part of it. Logging, blogging, and jogging.

If I feel well enough on Saturday, I'll run my five-and-a-half-mile race and go back to my mother's for the first Mother's Day without Dad. There may be more tears. But I want to accept them as the expression of what I can't say with words. As a part of the healing process. Poor food choices work against that. So that's not going to be on the program.

I did run my race, and I did go to my mother's. I thought my cold would prevent me, but I felt better and that changed my mind. I found that I could change my brain too.

PLASTICITY OF THE BRAIN
May 14, 2014

This concept is what is helping me right now. I can change my brain. I have brought back piano pieces from obscure memory. It takes a lot of practice. Sometimes I can only play a few measures before a mess up, but I've done it before. If I keep at it, there's a breakthrough, and more comes back. Sometimes it needs a little break for consolidation. Maybe a little sleep or rest. But in time, I've brought the music back to performance mode again.

I will get me back to performance mode again. I'll use my tools the way they work for me. I might mess up some, but I won't be giving up. There's a difference between messing up and giving up. And I'm not giving up. I'm still practicing. I will be back

I seem to have gotten sidetracked by some things recently. I think my old reactions to stress and grief and fears and even happiness were dredged up from somewhere I'd forgotten to clean out. Or maybe I didn't even know it was there to clean out. Whatever. The cleaning out of that part is being worked. And the practicing of me being me is happening. It's a matter of choosing to keep focused on what really matters.

Even though I have addictive tendencies when I'm under the influence of sugar, I can change my brain by using my tools and making the right choices and reinforcing the benefits of making those choices. I've done it before. And with regular practice, I'll get it back. To performance mode.

When I felt like I had a breakthrough in understanding, I found there was usually a follow-on.

AND THEN WHAT?
May 15, 2014

I had a lightbulb moment during a sugar problem. I became aware that I was thinking of what I would indulge in next even before I had finished the current indulgence. The thought was: Where will this "and then what" end? And I was scared, because I couldn't see it ending. I could only see me gaining weight. Not making lifetime weigh-in for May. Not making the June health goal for an insurance incentive bonus. Being depressed. Alienating people. Not fitting into my clothes. Blowing up like a self-inflatable life preserver. Except it wasn't to preserve life. It was looking more like a diet disaster.

But then I realized I could end it if I chose to. Back to my tools. I've proven what works for me. And when I do it, I am healthy even if my weight isn't in a prescribed place right away. There's a sense of control in doing what works. I can take care of me and, in turn, be able to take care of people I love. I can accept care from them too.

Three meals a day. No grazing. Greatly reduced sugar. A multivitamin. Tracking my food. Moving. Blogging my thoughts. Sleeping enough. Drinking water. Reading blogs and commenting. Drinking more water. Writing a blog post. And reading comments.

And then what?

More of the same. More (een) of the sane.

This next post was on the first anniversary of my dad's stroke. It was also my twenty-ninth wedding anniversary. I don't remember what was going on to prompt this topic, but it's okay.

IT'S OK. ONLY KIND.
May 25, 2014

I do not need to beat myself up over what I ate the day before yesterday or the day before that. But I can beef myself up, I suppose. Especially if it's more lean. And as far as that goes, I could beet myself up. Beets are good. Choosing to eat things that make me feel bad is bad enough. It isn't helpful to me when I get all down and depressed about it. Kindness is much more powerful than continuing the battle against me.

That punishment thing reminds me of something I thought of a few days ago: If someone is sensitive to gluten and eats it anyway, does it mean they are a gluten for punishment? The whole idea of eating to punish oneself is a bit preposterous when I think about it. It sounds like it might be great fodder for a therapy session. There's a certain contradiction of ideas at work regarding a binge on comfort foods.

Maybe it's just a mistaken interpretation of comfort. Does a bowl of sweetened whipped cream equal comfort? Does a cream-filled donut provide loving care? Or a whole bag of dates from Sam's Club? Perhaps there's a millisecond of time when my brain has a heightened sense of well-being. But the aftereffects are: give me more. And the effects on my mind, my skin, my clothes, and my relationships are not good.

To get mad at myself for making poor choices doesn't help me make better choices. What usually happens in that scenario is making worse choices. Like knowingly eating terrible food even when I'm not hungry. Even when my clothes are already getting tighter.

What helps me make better choices is to notice how I feel physically and emotionally after I eat anything. Good or bad. And instead of reinforcing the bad and feeling worse, I choose to work on good and feeling better. Because that's what matters. It's OK. Only Knowing. It's part of a learning process that is vital to continuing on this journey that is lifetime. My writing is a big part of that. I'm eating kind food today. The kind that comforts my health and makes it really feel better. I feel better in my mind. It really is OK.

Almost two months later, I was still working at it.

LiViNG MY PLAN. LOViNG MY PLAN. NOT LEAViNG MY PLAN.
July 14, 2014

I am on day six of my back-to-normal routine. The one that works for me and my brain. The one that helps me control my sugar addiction. I will not say that I have sugar addiction beat. I think I will always be a recovering addict. Because it doesn't take much to let it be a problem. I'm just soaking in this feeling of control. I don't crave the sugar. I crave the control. I am on high alert. Working three meals a day. Keeping sugar at bay. Exercising my way and writing word play.

I got a walk in this morning. And a Jazzercise class. Three meals are done. I wrote a blog post and erased it. And then wrote this. It's not very exciting. But it's a record of survival. And thankfulness. Tomorrow, I will get my license renewed. It's the first time in years that I will not wish that I'd lost fifty pounds before it was time to renew it. I did that, and more, a couple of years ago. And it's still valid. Most of it. Enough of it to look like I'm not overweight.

The next day I will turn fifty-two. I could find someone born in 1964 and do the whole, "How old are you? Fifty? Yeah, I'm fifty-two!" The thing where it sounds like I'm saying, "I'm fifty too." But I don't think I'll bother. I'm not having a problem with my age. Because I feel better at this age than when I was forty-two. Maybe even thirty-two. I'm living it. Healthy.

As I continued my living, I continued to encounter life. Road trips became a big part of my life. I was watching for signs on the highway and in my healthy journey too.

SHOULDER DROP-OFF AREA
August 17, 2014

My latest road trip was to help my oldest daughter with her move to a different city. One of the road signs we passed was "Shoulder Drop-Off Area." It was obviously a road construction warning, but my daughter and I found it amusing. Done with the cold shoulder? Drop it off here! Or something like that.

But then I texted a friend who likes interesting signs. (She has in her collection "Hilltop Marina" and "Handicap Area - No Standing" and "Lake Pond Brook." They're all signs with a lot of wonders.) As I typed the word *shoulder*, I started to second-guess the spelling and I looked it up. Then I looked again and saw shoulder differently. Should-er. Sort of like "should have" with a vernacular twist. I should-er done this, or I should-er done that. It fits right in with my observations and ramblings of a recovering sugar addict.

I had another learning experience this week on my road trip. The outbound trip was in a car. Six hours of driving the first day and twelve hours of driving the second day. My strategy was to keep with my three-meals-a-day, no-grazing, greatly-reduced-sugar eating plan. I had a plan to drink plenty of water, seltzer, and unsweetened tea. I didn't have opportunity to track or blog online. The drinking part of the plan was tied into exercising every couple of hours to use the facilities at rest areas. It worked.

But then we got to our destination. I should-er kept water and seltzer and tea nearby while I was helping with the move-in, but that all dropped off in the area of too much to do in too little time. I should-er paid more attention. Especially since it was eighty-six degrees with a real feel of ninety-five. I had packed my running gear, and I should-er used it but there was no time. I got my exercise hauling boxes and bags and pieces of furniture across a yard and upstairs to my daughter's second-floor apartment.

I flew back to my home state yesterday. I had a lot of waiting time at the airport. And although I did some walking around, I should-er done more. I think that dropped off because I was so tired. I should-er gotten some water to drink. But I dropped off my resolve in the Starbucks line and got an iced chai. I should-er dumped it out when I realized it was way too sweet for me. But I didn't. And so went the day. I should-er stopped at that. But I didn't. It was kind of wild.

My connecting flight was through Philadelphia. The gate area I waited at was for puddle-jumper service—tiny little planes with propellers. I heard an announcement requesting a volunteer to take a later flight so they could be light enough to take off! It was a weight-restricted flight—not based on the number of people in seats. I started feeling like I should-er skipped the cranberry orange scone and the curried chicken sandwich and the iced mocha. But my plane wasn't overweight.

The woman in the seat next to me didn't fit with the armrest down. And her seat belt didn't fasten around her. It could have been me a few years ago. She chose water to drink. I wondered if she might be working on better health. I wish her the best.

I was thankful that my row (the last one in the plane) had empty seats in it. I moved over to the middle seat and had the most leg room I've ever had on a flight. It was open all the way to the cockpit door. Eight rows and the galley! I made it home safe and sound. (Engine noise *and* flying over Long Island Sound!)

Now I am shouldering the burden of my choices. But instead of angst and regret and diving into more things that I should avoid, I'm learning. My next trip is to Jacksonville, Florida. Maybe I'll find a sign at the Department of Animal Control: The Pound Drop-Off Area.

By the time summer was over, I had logged thousands of miles and thousands of words. But just as important as editing pictures for a travelogue, I've worked at selecting the best words for my book.

NOW. MiXiNG iT UP.

September 5, 2014

I've been on road trips for most of the summer. Some of the time, I've felt good about my food choices and care of my health. But since the middle of August, I've been tripping up on all kinds of hazards.

I've learned a lot. I already knew that pride goes before a fall. (Summer does too, for that matter.) I also learned that Waffle House goes before a fall. It's not an excuse. But it has taken a while to get my seat belt buckled again. Fortunately, it still buckles without an extender. Although I've covered a lot of ground, I'm not running a cover-up. I OWN this, and that's part of a victory I WON.

In mid-July, I traveled with a second cousin who was visiting from California. We drove more than a thousand miles in less than a week. I met her in Boston, and we covered bits of Massachusetts; New Hampshire; New York (including Letchworth Falls and Niagara Falls); Ontario, Canada (we walked there from New York); Connecticut; and Rhode Island (including lobster rolls and whole belly clams at the beach in Newport). I kept my eating to mealtimes. We did plenty of walking as well as talking. It was all good.

I spent several days in southern New Hampshire at an annual gathering. They were good days for my spirit and soul. They weren't food-focused. I felt well cared for and loved. I kept my natural eating to mealtimes and got a good amount of hill walking in.

Directly after my time in New Hampshire, I helped my oldest daughter drive to the St. Louis area. She moved there for work and school. I kept my eating plan fairly in control until I was waiting for my flight home to Connecticut. I reined it in after a couple of days of craziness.

I had a week at home helping my youngest daughter get ready to move to Florida for school. We had another annual gathering to attend in New York just before we left. My time in New York was great. I was busy in the mornings, and I kept my breakfasts to a plant-based protein powder shake with coconut oil and chia seeds added in. It kept me until lunchtime, and I felt in control of my eating the rest of the day too.

My husband and daughter and I drove our packed van and our daughter's packed car to Florida in two days. I did most of the van driving. I listened to an audiobook about food addiction. And then to another book about fat, sugar, and salt and the food industry's use of them to increase sales. I drank lots of water and unsweetened tea. And I had to stop every couple of hours to use a restroom. That was the first day.

The second day began at Waffle House with indecision about what to order. I should have gone with two poached eggs. But when it came to actually placing the order, I got a combo breakfast. It had more points than a compass, I think. The eggs would have covered north, south, east, and west. But what I ordered covered all the points in between too. The rest of my time involved *fats* food and the onset of grazing.

My husband flew back home for work. I stayed in Florida for a few days to help my daughter get settled. And then I drove home. I had several overnight stops with relatives. My mother flew to North Carolina to be with me in Virginia for a few days and then be company for the rest of the trip. I'll just say that I didn't eat like a healthy person.

I thought I would just get back to my normal, healthy, thin-person eating style, but reality proved that wrong. I'm not quite done with my road trips. But I am done with the craziness. NOW. Negate Over Weight.

So I'm back to blogging. And logging. And I'll do some jogging. It might not be a straight line back, but I'm on my way. And then I'll be on my weigh. As a side effect of using the tools that work for me.

I OWN this. (Official Wake-up Nudge) But *now*, I'm Working On Necessary things. Looks like I WON. It's ongoing.

In my travels, I encountered speed bumps, but the one I liked the idea of the most was in Florida.

SPEED BUMPS AND MORE
September 13, 2014

When I was in Florida, I stayed with a good friend. We were chatting about her kitchen and how she wants to remodel it. One thing that's going to go is the flooring. The house is on a slab, and for some reason, the flooring buckles every once in a while. She said that one time she had a speed bump in front of her fridge! They fixed it, but I thought it was a marvelous idea!

My friend reminisced about a conversation we had back in May. She'd been on a special detoxing plan, but a baby shower got in her way. She had a tiny piece of cake and something else that didn't fit into her eating plan. I suggested that she simply own it and move on. And she did. I was pleased that my comment had helped her. And more pleased that she brought it up in conversation, because I needed to hear it for me. And do it.

I am simply owning this summer. The events were significant. That I succumbed to sugar shouldn't be the focus. My oldest daughter moved halfway across the country. My youngest daughter moved a similar distance, but south. I drove 4,500 or so miles, and much of it was by myself. I came home to an empty nest. My mother had surgery. Another of my dad's cousins died. My son and his wife are expecting a baby girl in January. It was my first summer without a dad.

Sugar took its toll, but I'm tired of paying. I woke up this morning with arthritic-type pains in my hands and my back. Those are pains that I got rid of three years ago when I ditched sugar.

Each night this week, I've been done with sugar. But each day, at some point, I've succumbed again. And again. Today, with the aches and pains, I'm done again. Sugar isn't a speed bump to my success, it's a blockade. And it has to go. I'm going to reclaim my mental clarity. I'm writing a blog post instead of eating between meals. I'm going to win. Using the tools. Logging (my food) and blogging (my mood). Jogging will come. In time.

The human brain has a wonderful capacity for storing information. My ability to retrieve it is called remembering, but sometimes I seem to forget how to do it.

REMEMBERING. RE: MEMBER
September 14, 2014

I am a member of WW because I use the tracking tools to record my food. I use the blogging tools to record my mood and to connect with other people who are using this tool.

I am remembering why I joined the online program in January 2012. It wasn't to be on a diet. It was to use the tools on my journey to good health. And I'm remembering that the journey doesn't stop.

I am a few pounds above goal weight right now. I had to pay a monthly fee to keep using the tools, because my free eTools ran out. Sugar is the main culprit. But maybe not completely. I think I got into a place where I paid attention to what people were saying about how I looked. Fabulous. Wonderful. Wow. The comments were from people who hadn't seen me since I lost close to ninety pounds. They hadn't seen me at my lowest weight. The weight where I could wear size-four clothes and still breathe.

A friend of mine was commenting this weekend about how wonderful it was that I was still slender after three years. I'd kept the weight off, and that's really something. But I let her know that some of the weight had come back, and I needed to get rid of it again. She said I still looked good—did I feel good? And I had to say I didn't feel good. And she understood. Eating right is about feeling good. The weight loss is a side effect.

I'm remembering. And it's good to be back at it.

I liked the idea of shrinking my body size and also "shrinking" my mind. It was amateur therapy, I suppose, but sometimes I did it in prose.

SHRiNKiNG
September 15, 2014

I noticed fairly early that blogging was a form of therapy. Instead of going to a shrink, I was writing my way to healthy. That was the write way for me, and it worked. But there has been a relapse that needs more thought. So here I am trying to shrink myself again.

I think this post has to do with body image—as in, I feel gross, therefore I must look gross. And then someone says how fabulous I look. This happened multiple times over the summer. Some of the people hadn't seen me at my healthiest. And others hadn't seen me since I'd lost so much weight starting in 2011.

I got back from a long road trip this summer and weighed less than I thought I would. I had derailed in my resolve to not eat between meals. I'd eaten more fast food than usual. And I hadn't gotten as much exercise. I didn't feel good. But the number on the scale wasn't too bad. Just a few pounds above goal.

I had every opportunity to get back in control with logging, jogging, and blogging. But I didn't seem to have enough umph to really want to do it. I needed umph to go with my try, and although there were a couple of good days, I didn't string them together. Instead, I seemed determined to eat everything not good for me. And if it wasn't available, I'd make it.

I managed to rein things in a few times. Like the day I threw out most of a double batch of fudge that wasn't setting up. Another day I threw out an almost-full can of whipped cream. That was the day I threw out the carton of ice cream and cleared the cupboard of all the baking mixes for cakes and brownies.

So technically, it could have been a lot worse. But it wasn't good. It was ridiculous. I would do green smoothies for breakfast and a protein-rich lunch. And dive head first into a box of granola with half-and-half midafternoon. (I finally threw out the box of granola.) My weight was fluctuating five to seven pounds down and up. Diet mode. Scale focused. And then not a shred of caring.

I think part of it was the sugar-clouded thought process combined with the number sugar does on my impulse controls. What people were saying (fabulous) wasn't matching up to what the scale was saying and what my body was saying (flabu-lousy). I seemed to be on a tear to end anyone even dreaming of saying fabulous. My sugar addiction will use any and all reasons or possibilities to make poor food choices.

I felt lousy and thought I looked lousy. But the big reason I felt lousy was my food choices. I know this because in January 2012, I weighed fifty pounds more than I do right now and felt great because I had started eating right. I was using the tools, and I was feeling in control.

Last night, someone said I looked fabulous. I had just gotten back from a workout. And perhaps she thought it would be encouraging to me. Or maybe she really thought I looked good. Anyway, what I realized is this: People are entitled to their opinions. But they don't live in my skin. Flattery doesn't have to lead to fattery.

I have to pay attention to what my body is saying. Not my sugar addiction. I can't let the scale determine how I eat, either. A quick drop in weight from diet-like eating is not a way for me to feel healthy. Diets don't work for me.

What works for me is using the WW tools with the guidelines I adapted from *Potatoes Not Prozac*. Three meals a day. No grazing. Enough protein. Enough water. Good food. Not diet food. Exercise. A multivitamin. I have had a good day today. Even with a headache from sugar withdrawal. Or maybe I should say especially with a headache from sugar withdrawal. Because I feel hope. For caution and control.

Lifetime crops up in my manuscript quite often. I think it's because that's the total picture every day.

LiFETiME STUFF
October 23, 2014

It's a daily thing. And I did it today.

A challenge for lunch
Not with great ease
I avoided dessert
With a "none for me, please."

I oohed over smell
And the artful sight
But explained why I wouldn't
Take even one bite.

The hostess was kind
And let me decline
With nary a fuss
And I was fine.

Some of the gaps between the posts are because of editing. Others are because nothing was there. The following post explains a gap. Rather than being upset, I'm learning from it. I need to write often.

BLOGGING AND MORE (EEN)—BAM!
December 1, 2014

I haven't posted for a few weeks. And it shows. I've tried, and I've cried. My "This Time Last Year" post was too painful to finish. I started it just before Thanksgiving and couldn't manage to write the "This Time This Year" part of it. Last year, my dad was with us. This year, he is a memory. Last year, I was in control of my food, my moods, and my moves. This year, not so much. Maybe it's a part of the grieving process? Or not.

And so, I've had another learning experience. The relapse. The feeling lousy. The aches and pains. The recognition of closet eating. The realization that the next mouthful is the focus, not the family. The stark reality that clothes don't fit. The grumpies. The sadness. The lack of control.

Pulling out the Learning Experience from BLAME turns it into BAM! The simply owning. The soldiering on. The stop overeating. But not the start over. Because I didn't quit. (I'm not focused on blame. Because I see it as b-lame. It makes me limp and feel like a wimp. It feels a bit like a crutch that I really don't need. I want my steps firm to succeed!)

Thanksgiving this year was at my son and daughter-in-law's house in Maine. We got there at the beginning of a snowstorm on Wednesday. It was wonderful to see them, our sweet little grandson, and signs of our granddaughter's impending arrival. Thursday morning at three o'clock, the power went off. Fortunately, they had a coal stove and a good supply of coal. And fortunately, they have a gas stove with a range top that works with a manual start.

I got a bit of exercise with shoveling and playing with my grandson in the foot of snow the storm had delivered. And then there was the question of what to do for Thanksgiving dinner. There were several options, including going to another location. But the one we settled on was for me to carve the thawed raw turkey and turn it into stir-fry meat for a new twist on Thanksgiving dinner.

At this point, I was doing great with my no grazing and staying away from sugar. We had brought lots of vegetables and fruit to go with the meal. And then someone decided to toast some pecans on the coal stove. I thought I would resist tasting them. I know what they taste like, and I also know that I don't stop eating them once I start. I proved that once again. And my resolve got stuck in a snow bank. Or maybe a NO bank. I was saying no to my healthy self, and the addiction was awake.

The good news out of this, though, is that my turkey stir-fry was really good. It wasn't free range, it was gas range. And even though we had no power, it was loaded with power foods. And several thought it was a better than a traditional turkey dinner.

I turned the leftovers into turkey curry with some coconut milk and curry powder. I boiled the remainder of the meat on the carcass and managed to make two quarts of turkey vegetable rice soup and a southwestern-style turkey rice casserole to freeze for easy meals when they need them. I get a thrill out of cooking creatively, and I really appreciate that my daughter-in-law let me do it!

The other good news is that it only took a couple of days (not months or years) to get to the other side of the learning experience with a renewed BAM (Be Aware, Maureen! Or is it Be Awesome, Maureen!). I am feeling empowered again. I can be in control when I'm using the tools. Logging my foods, blogging my moods, and jogging my moves. I don't want the consequences that come with sugar. Wheat has joined the ranks of sugar as a trigger of addictive behavior, and I'm feeling glad to say no to it once again. Thankful to know. And thankful to know what to do about it. Thankful to have a place to talk about it. To myself. And anyone who might want to listen.

I ran three miles yesterday, and I did a Jazzercise class this morning. I roasted a large turkey in my oven overnight and picked the meat and boiled the bones this morning. I have some health-friendly meals and soups to make for today and also to freeze for easy future meals.

It's good.

Too many times, my focus would be on what I did wrong. But there was a lot to notice that was right.

SOMETHING I AM DOING RIGHT
December 3, 2014

I have been having a chopped romaine salad for lunch this week. A whole head of romaine (the kind that comes in a package of six at Sam's); a hard-boiled egg, chopped; one-quarter of an avocado, chunked; four pepperoncini, sliced; four ounces of roasted turkey, chopped; one tablespoon regular mayonnaise; and salt and pepper. Today I added a can of drained beets with a drizzle of balsamic vinegar. Twice, I sliced four black olives in the mix. And twice, I added about a half a cup of pomegranate seeds.

It looks good, and it is good. It takes a long time to eat. The choppedness of it makes it impossible to wolf down. I will sheepishly add that I tend to eat too fast. Yum-*mee*! (That's what my nineteen-month-old grandson says.)

I'm also doing something write. I'm blogging my way through some challenging moments. There are a lot of them today, but while I'm writing, I'm not eating. And I'm exercising my brain and fingers. And now, to quote my grandson again, "All done!"

Where to focus is the answer to some questions.

REPEAT
December 4, 2014

I was thinking about eating and exercising. And I think a little confusion in the picture could lead to a problem. Reps of eating instead of reps of exercising. Rep eats. Fork lifts instead of bicep curls. And then I thought about a different way to look at the word. Re: Peat. Something about fuel. But that's not my turf.

All corniness aside, I was thinking of what my weight-loss journey or whole-life journey has been. Finding what works for me, using the tools effectively, and then slipping up.

Historically (or hysterically), I've thought of that repetition as always ending on the slipping-up part. But I think it's a good idea for me to see the getting-back-up part. The continuing part. The not-quitting part. Even when there's a slipup. Because I do get back up. I use the same tools I used at the beginning. Logging, jogging, and blogging. My good health comes back. I feel like myself again. And my weight takes care of itself.

Lather, rinse, repeat. Clean again. Blather, sense, repeat.

I didn't need to use the auto club, AAA, while I was on my road trips, but I found a lot of help for figurative planning and roadside assistance in case of emergency in my personal AAA.

DOING WHAT WORKS FOR HEALTHY. AAA.
January 3, 2015

I do stuff every day. And it all works. But sometimes it works against me. Sugar works against my impulse controls. Sitting around works against my fitness goals. Those two combined work against my mind. (And that sounds like a poem of the rhyming kind.)

This healthy thing. It works for me. But sometimes my mind works against it. When I use the blogging tool, the tracking tool, and the guidelines from *Potatoes Not Prozac*, my mind comes around and helps work the healthy thing. I am now in year four of this concept, and I continue to learn about myself.

I'm thinking about **A**wareness, **A**cceptance, and **A**daptability. My triple A. In order to know I need help, I have to be **A**ware. I am very aware that sugar is a problem for me. That is not enough, though. I have to accept this and understand it is just a part of me. Not good or bad. Just is. And to do me justice, I need to accept the parameters that help me manage. Logging, jogging, and blogging. Adaptability. I can adapt. I adapted off close to ninety pounds and kept them off for months.

As long as I keep aware of my sugar problem and accept it, I can live with adaptations that work for my good. Trip planning and roadside assistance.

Coming to grips and holding on.

JUST IS VS. JUSTICE
January 4, 2015

It's a slippery slope when my mind tries to reason out what's fair. It actually turns out to be a circus—going around and rounder. Some things just aren't fair. They just are. Just is. Sometimes a meal isn't fare. Just is served. And it can turn into a circus complete with a fat lady. Me. If I don't pay attention to what just is.

I once heard a story about a woman who didn't like a picture of herself. She told the photographer, "It doesn't do me justice." The photographer replied, "Lady, what you need is mercy." Whether that is funny or not doesn't matter to me. I like the idea of mercy. And the thought that came along with that is derived from my high school French. *Merci* very much.

When I can accept what just is, and feel thankful that I have a way to manage it, things are good. I feel good. And (I flatter myself) look good. My "just is" happens to be sugar addiction. And when I ignore that, it's just ice. Slipping and falling. Mercy. Another chance. And I'm thankful I can be thinkful again.

The past few days have been tough. And they could get tougher. But not because of sugar. I'm aware. I'm accepting. I'm adapting. Because I'm an addict that has to apply the A game. The triple-A game. Awareness, Acceptance, and Adaptability. All the time. It just is.

Sometimes there are no excuses because there isn't any need or reason for them!

NO EXCUSES
January 9, 2015

A happy day. My granddaughter was born early this morning. My son has a daughter. My grandson has a sister. My daughter-in-law is amazing. All are doing well. The pictures are beautiful. I won't get to meet her until next week. That's a good reason to keep doing what works for me.

With all the excitement of a starting a road trip, there was an excitement in knowing it would end at home.

HOME
January 14, 2015

It is good to be back. The car is unpacked, a load of laundry is halfway done, supper was made and eaten, and my suitcase is put away.

Yesterday, we had a hotel breakfast. In times past, I would have had a feeding frenzy with the sausage gravy, pastries, eggs, coffee with hot chocolate, and fresh waffles. Even if it didn't taste great. Because that's what I, under the influence of sugar, would do. But yesterday, I mixed a packet of plain oatmeal with banana slices, a packet of cream cheese (I wanted some fat), and hot water. It was tasty. I also had one hard-boiled egg. It wasn't so tasty, but it was protein. I had my multivitamin. And I was done with eating until lunchtime.

Lunchtime was a Wendy's baked potato with a small order of chili on top. I followed that with a couple of clementines, and that was that until supper. I kept hydrated with water and the occasional unsweetened tea.

The only time I ate between meals was a planned and defined snack this morning while my daughter was sleeping.

I had one cashew every mile for twenty miles. It took the hungry and bored feeling away. And I was so pleased to prove that I could do it. I tracked it when I stopped driving. I don't think I've ever eaten nuts one at a time. One handful at a time and when I was done, the can would have been empty instead of almost full.

I have more to write. But not right now. It's enough to say I'm home. I'm still using AAA. I'm Aware that there are dangers lurking after a successful experience. I'm Accepting that fact. I'm Adapting. I have a plan for tomorrow, and it's good.

The more common phrase is happily ever after, but I decided I liked it mixed up as an aid to keep me in order on my journey.

HAPPY AFTER EVER

January 18, 2015

I like the idea of happy after ever. Because it's still happening. The days after my trip continue to be clean and happy. I'm working my tools the way I worked them when I started this journey in January 2012.

I've had some sad moments this past week. But they haven't been about food or sugar. I'm remembering last year at this time. My father was dying. It wasn't an easy experience. But I got through it with a lot of help from faith, family, and friends. No sugar added.

So sometimes life isn't so happy. Perhaps it could be called happen. Life happens. Happy and sad and in between. From my experience, the sad happens in a better way when I am not controlled by sugar. So does the happy.

This weekend is the first anniversary of my dad's passing. I still miss him. But I am thankful for so many wonderful memories and his influence. This weekend I met my granddaughter for the first time. She is precious, and I look forward to making special memories with her. And I hope to be a good influence for her. Without sugar.

ONGOING CONCLUSION

The End Is an Illusion but Not at All Confusion

With a continuing story, it's hard to find a stopping place. Every moment becomes history sooner or later. But there would be no history books if the historian waited for his story to be done.

HiSTORY. THAT'S A WRAP!

January 29, 2015

We had a snowstorm this week. Well, it was officially a blizzard, I think. Lots of snow and wind. We got around twenty inches of light, fluffy snow. The drifts were high. It's not prehistoric anymore. It's part of history. The sun has come out. The driveway is clear. We're back in business. Until this next "prehistoric" storm arrives. (I've decided that prehistoric is just another way of thinking about the future!)

What I really wanted to write about isn't history. It's mystory. That looks a bit like mystery. But there's no mystery in my story. I know what's going on. And I know what went on. I started grazing last week. A little relaxing of my plan. And *wham*. Well, not that fast, but quick enough, I dipped into more and more between meals. I excused myself at first by saying, "Well, at least I'm not eating wheat or sugar." And then it was, "Well, I'm not eating wheat." And I was stuck in the drift. A sugar-high drift.

This thing that is mystory involves sugar addiction. When I don't use my tools, I join the ranks of the fools. I fool myself into thinking it's not so bad. Then I feel like a cad. And expand instead of shrinking.

This morning I started a new detox. After nearly a month of clean. The worst of the sugar storm raged for a day. Completely. Out. Of. Control. This morning, my thoughts came in rhyme. It works best out loud.

I was heading back
to the ranks of obese
How and why did that happen?
A slip and a fall
and that is not all
But I'm starting to feel like
Rappin'.

There's a certain rhythm I find
That helps me get off my behind
Spurs me to action
Gives me some traction
To hope and want to be kind
To myself.
Resolve's off the shelf
I'm working my spiels
Not spinning my wheels.
Using my tools with my special rules.
Oh, yeah.
It's not a broken record
I say it for the record
I'm bookin' t'ward success
Getting out
of my own mess
Cut the candy wrapper
I'm back
More E'en the Rapper!

It's about shrinking myself. An ongoing process. Being aware and able
to care. Living with sugar addiction. It's a lifetime thing. It's what I do.
I dare. I'm possible!

AND THEN WHAT HAPPENED?

Going On And Living

I had to pick an end point for my book, but I still write almost every day. It's part of what I do to stay in control. I've stayed away from sugar for months now. I'm managing my weight. My thoughts are clear, and my moods don't swing with drama. I still struggle with addiction, but I've been noticing the warning signs earlier. A slipup is more likely to be grazing, but not with sugar. When I realize I've gotten lax with tracking and notice I'm not paying as much attention to the scale, it's a red flag to polish my tools by using them more. I'm including a blog post from just before I submitted my final revisions.

PiCTURE THiS
October 6, 2015

I posted two pictures recently. They're before and after pictures in the sense of sugar and no sugar.

In the before picture, I am laughing, but I am also hurting. It was June 2011. We had gone for a walk on the Marginal Way in Ogunquit after my son got married farther up the Maine coast. My feet hurt from my new, shiny shoes, and my body hurt from wearing too much fat. I was resolved that I would not let my shape—body and mind—get in the way of my son's wedding. And I think I was successful. I did not focus on myself. I let the cameras snap without trying to hide. I chatted and visited and kept busy doing the things the mother of the groom does. Or at least this mother of that groom does. But underneath, I was hurting in my body and in my mind. I now know that sugar was the biggest cause of that.

The other picture is from last week. I'm more than four years older, more than sixty pounds lighter, and pretty much pain-free. I know I was tired in that picture, but I wasn't spending extra energy trying to look happy. I was happy. I was helping my daughter with her photography class homework. I drove; she snapped pictures. And when we stopped at the banks of the Connecticut River, she turned her camera on me.

I will not claim that everything is roses without sugar. Or maybe I can. Roses have thorns, and sometimes they hurt. I think I can say my life is more real without sugar. I can experience all the shades of emotion and feelings without trying to eat my way through them. I can feel without trying to numb myself with food. I have learned that nothing is better with a sugar hangover.

I know there are many people who feel like what I've done with sugar is impossible for them to do. I know what that feeling is like. I used to think it was impossible too, until I read the back cover of *Potatoes Not Prozac* and felt a glimmer of hope. That glimmer turned into a flame of purpose to be aware of how I was feeling, accept that I had a problem with sugar, and adapt my lifestyle to feel better. It turned into logging, jogging, and blogging. Which turned into me. The real me. I'm possible.

You are possible too! It takes awareness, acceptance, and adapting. Find tools that work for you, and use them. To good health!

POINTING THE WAY TO RESOURCES

A Starting Point to Finding the Right Tools for You

If you are feeling inspired to start your own "I'm Possible" tool collection, congratulations! I've listed some of the resources that I use. They might be helpful for you. If you're actively using a tool and it isn't working for you, find a different way to use it or just get rid of it. Perhaps there's a better tool to help you be successful. There's value in knowing what doesn't work! Best wishes on your "I'm possible" journey!

1. *Potatoes Not Prozac: A Natural Seven-Step Dietary Plan to Stabilize the Level of Sugar in Your Blood, Control Your Cravings and Lost Weight, and Recognize How Foods Affect the Way You Feel* by Kathleen DesMaisons Ph.D.

This is the book that helped me understand that I could change impossible to I'm possible. The edition I read was from 1998. However, she has written several revisions since then. Dr. DesMaisons also has a website (http://staging.radiantrecovery.com/) that has additional information about living with sugar sensitivity.

2. WW International Weight Watchers International, now known as WW, weightwatchers reimagined (http://www.weightwatchers.com)

I joined WW online as a way to track my food and blog my feelings based on what I learned in *Potatoes Not Prozac*. I also wanted to use their points system to make sure I ate enough to lose weight (if I could), and that's what happened. I wasn't so much "on" WW as I was using their tools to work for me. It made all the difference. WW has changed dramatically since I started using their tools. They changed their points system and eliminated blogging. It's not my favorite tool anymore, but it might work for you.

3. *Holiday Detox* by Joy Bauer (http://www.today.com/health/new-year-new-you-joy-bauers-simple-detox-diet-2D80555514)

My husband and I had previously used this plan to get back to clean eating after holiday indulgences. It took the guesswork out of what to eat for a few days. I found that it fit with my use of *Potatoes Not Prozac* and WW. I don't use it very often, but I'm glad I have it when I need it.

4. *Healing Back Pain: The Mind-Body Connection* by John E. Sarno, MD

I mentioned this book when I wrote about my half marathon experience. I found it to be a great awareness tool. Pain (and hunger) are not always physical.

5. www.maureenaliprandi.com

Visit me at my website!

6. www.impossiblejourneyblog.wordpress.com

This is where I've been blogging since WW discontinued their blogging community. There are many places to record your thoughts in a supportive community setting. Find what works for you and do it!

Printed in the United States
By Bookmasters